I AM
Girl Power

I AM GIRL POWER

KATIE CROSS

CONTENTS

I Am Girl Power

Chick Lit

Cover designed by Jenny Zemanek with Seedlings Online

Published by KC Writing.

To Megan Gray. You are the girl power in me.

1

STERILE BREAKS

Sweatpants, flip-flops, and a braid never let me down.

Despite the luxury of my boyfriend's elegant, low-lighted dinner gala unfurling around me, I couldn't stop thinking about my comfortable sweats. My dress itched in all the wrong places, digging into my ribs like teeth. The arch of my left foot spasmed. I gritted my teeth and smiled through it for the tenth time.

With a sigh of resignation, I searched for Nathan again. Empty chairs ringed the tables laden with glittering crystal and vases of orchids. The floral scent gave me a headache. How he managed to mingle so effortlessly, I'd never understand.

Luckily, no one paid attention to me. I slipped my left heel off and groaned when my tense foot relaxed against the cool tile floor.

Heaven.

"Ah! Megan. There you are. I've been looking everywhere for you."

Nathan swept up to my side, setting a hand on the small of my back. He reminded me of a hawk. Shrewd. Sharp. Intelligent to a fault. With his straight nose and strong features, he looked like a Greek god.

"Where've you been?" I asked.

"Working the room."

Nathan could mingle with a school of sharks and still cut a business deal. His studious gaze hadn't stopped scanning the room, but the edges of his lips twitched upward. Something must be happening.

"What's going on?" I drawled, popping my right heel off and suppressing the urge to toss the heels into a punch fountain. Instead of rubbing my feet—I had some sense of social decorum—I wiggled my newly freed toes.

Nathan nodded toward the other side of the room where a lanky man with wisps of thin hair around his temples lingered near the punch bowl.

"See him?" he asked.

"Yes."

"That's the CEO, Marshall Grant. I just spoke with him."

A prickle of intuition raised the hair on the back of my neck. *CEO?* Nathan had been salivating over a promotion ever since we started dating six weeks ago. "Nate," I said, eyeing him. "Do you have something important to tell me?"

His composure broke, and he gave me his signature, sparkling smile that buckled my knees.

"Oh, nothing big. Just a little promotion. To Director." He paused. "In *New York City*."

I squealed. He threw his arms around me, swept me off my feet, and spun me in a circle. Once he set me down, I clutched his shoulders.

"Really?"

"Really."

"Nate!" I smacked his shoulder. "Great job! You've been working forever for this."

He ran a hand through his hair. His perfect locks skewed to the left in the most adorable way. "This is huge. Megs, I can't tell you. This is ... Titanic if it never hit an iceberg. Atlantis if it never sunk."

Neither of those things would have been legends without their terrific failures, but I let that go.

"Congratulations!"

"There's so much to do. I'll be moving. Probably next week. Sooner? No. Tomorrow is just too soon. Although I could rent a hotel room..."

His voice trailed off in a mumble. A wave of exhaustion swept over me as the clock caught my gaze. One in the morning. My bed and my sweats and braless freedom called for me.

"Let's talk about this in your car," I said around a yawn, collecting my discarded heels. Maids crept across the room with trash bins. The lights dimmed. Nathan muttered as he followed my insistent tugs toward the elevator and through the parking garage, unaware that I walked barefoot. He jerked his head back and forth as if answering his own questions, and we slipped inside his cherry-red Mustang.

Fifteen silent minutes later, he pulled up in front of my townhouse but didn't turn the car off. The seatbelt slid across my shoulder with a hiss when I released it, reaching for the door handle. He stared at the odometer with a fixed gaze.

"Nate?" I asked. "You okay?"

He blinked, as if coming out of a daze, and frowned. "No. Well, yes. Meg, we need to talk."

"Talk?"

"I'm worried that ... I think this promotion will complicate things between us."

"Nate, we're both workaholics. Things are already complicated."

"This is different. Long-distance relationships suck."

"So do breakups."

He rolled his eyes. "Don't make this harder than it needs to be. I don't think this will work anymore."

This, he'd said. What did *this* mean? My heart beat a heavy staccato in my ribs as the ugly truth wormed into my brain. No way. No *way* was he breaking up with me this evening.

"Whoa, Nate. Don't do this. Not on a whim. Listen, long-distance can suck, but it can be fun in its own way." *Mostly miserable.* "A-and visiting New York City will be fun!"

He scoffed. "Maybe for you."

My brow furrowed. "You don't want me to visit?"

He ran a hand through his hair. "It's not that. It's just going to be different. You're wonderful, Megan."

"Don't you dare—"

"But this promotion is going to be intense." He slipped into a robotic tone that made me want to fizzle all his circuits. "And I don't think it would be fair to you if I moved to New York City and buried myself in work. Besides, this never felt easy. You can't deny that."

"Good things are never easy!"

"But good relationships should be. We didn't have that *it* factor, you know? And I'm looking for *it*."

"What's *it*?"

"I don't know! I just know I'll feel it."

Oh, you're going to feel something in a minute. My nails dug into my palms. This relationship hadn't sunk yet. I could forgive this conversation. Forget the trapped fear in his eyes.

"Good relationships are hard work, Nate. Not even some magical *it* factor would change that."

He sighed and lifted his hands. "Meg, I'm ending this. I'm sorry. Thank you for all the time we've had together, but I think it's best we split ways."

A livid current of hurt and rage swept through me. "So that's it? You aren't even going to try?"

He tucked his chin to his chest and closed his eyes.

"No. We're done."

What about the good times? I wanted to say, although I couldn't think of one right then. *We're both career oriented. We both...*

My mind stuttered to a stop. Surely, we had something else in common. Some fantastic date to draw from? But my mind rang with empty silence. Besides, I'd been down this road before. Many, many times. Once he didn't want it, there was no reason to fight.

Sterile breaks like this were the hardest. Clean. Clinical. The lack of emotion left me feeling lost. I preferred sparks and livid shouting. Accusations hurt far less than passive silence.

"You'll be fine." He waved a hand through the air. "You're one of the strongest girls I've ever met. I know you'll meet someone who fits."

Be strong, then, Meg. That's what they all expect, isn't it? I clenched my fists. Girl power and all that.

"Right. Well. Best of luck!" I said brightly, reaching for the door handle. "Thanks for everything."

The words faltered only a little. He opened his mouth to say something, decided against it, and rested a hand on the back of my seat. To my delight, a hint of disappointment lingered on his downturned lips.

Yep, I wanted to say, I'm already over you.

"Uh ... yeah. See ya around, Meg."

I wouldn't come near you even if you paid me, lover boy.

His eyes followed me as I unlocked my door, shoulders straight and chin high. Once inside, I tossed the heels into a corner and ripped bobby pins out of my hair. I stormed through my townhouse, Medusa-style curls flowing in every direction as I peeled my dress off.

"Good riddance, Nathan," I yelled, tossing it out the open window. With outrage burning in my veins, I stalked to my bedroom to find the warmest pair of sweats I owned.

~

The World's Worst Breakup Excuses

- *"We have different life experiences. You're way ahead of me."*
- *"You're not really my type."*
- *"Let's get married. No? Okay. Let's break up."*
- *"You don't need me, and I want to be needed."*
- *"You do single so well!"*
- *"We didn't have that it factor, you know?"*

~

After lounging in my sweats all day Sunday—and avoiding my phone lest Nate call—I stepped into the Cardiac Intensive Care Unit on Monday morning with renewed determination.

Forget ex-boyfriends. Lose myself in work. Worked every time.

I stopped near the front desk and drew in a deep, relieved breath. The smell of alcohol and cleaning solution filled my nose with a comforting, familiar tang. At last, I could fall into the safety of nursing. Forget the cutting pain of rejection. Forget the lonely ache of my bruised heart.

Ah, work.

"You never let me down," I murmured to a bank of cardiac monitors as I swept by them, headed for the charge nurse's office with a spring in my step. Conversations buzzed in the air like human drones. A few bleary-eyed night shift nurses waved at me.

Work is always here, I thought. Nathan can dump me like all the rest of my failed relationships, but work never will. It always has my back.

"Here!" I announced as I slid into the charge nurse's office. "Is the floor busy today? I could use a crazy assignment."

Tami, charge nurse for the day shift, sat behind a computer. A clipboard, a stethoscope, and a copy of the patient assignments were splayed around her. Her left hand curled around a coffee mug like a sleepy cat. She regarded me with suspicion in her teardrop-shaped eyes.

"What happened to you?" she asked, straightening. "You look like the monster from a science fiction movie."

"Ah, Tami. You always did have a way with words."

She pointed to my feet. "Your shoes don't match. Why are you here? You're not on the schedule."

"Don't ask. Can I pick up an extra today?"

She blinked. "You came in here at 6:45 in the morning on the offhand chance I needed an extra nurse?"

"Yep."

"Don't you have a life?"

"Of course I have a life." I lifted both arms. "It's here at work! Just like yours."

Tami shook her head. "You're insane."

Desperate, I wanted to counter. It's a fine line.

"We always need an extra nurse these days," I said, perusing the patient assignments. "Give me the craziest assignment on the floor. Something that'll keep me running all day."

"No one requests that, you psycho. What happened?"

"Life," I muttered.

She glanced down at the papers with a rueful sigh. "That I can understand. I have five kids who insist on eating more than once a day. If our stupid CEO keeps running the hospital into the ground, it won't happen."

"Is that a *yes*?"

"No. But I think Karen may be looking for you. She asked whether you'd be here today."

"What did she want?"

"Dunno."

Why would my floor manager want to speak with me? I snapped my fingers. "I just took the test to get my certification in Critical Care Nursing. She probably got the results."

"Still hoping for a spot on the flight team?"

"Yep. Right on track, just as I've planned for the last six years." I tapped a picture of a helicopter and three of our nurses in flight suits. Working as a nurse on a helicopter required guts of steel; flight nurses were the tip of the sword. Skilled. Versatile. Talented. Flight nursing required intense training in life-saving procedures and flawless execution. Simply put, they dropped into ugly situations and saved lives while flying through the air. It had been my goal since I graduated nursing school.

Tami held up a fist. "Go get 'em, girl power."

I DUCKED out of the office, ignoring Tami's low grumbles about fewer vacation days, and headed toward the management alcove. A wedge of light spilled across the floor from the back-corner office.

"Karen?" I called, advancing into the room. "You in?"

"Come on in."

Karen, nurse manager for the CICU, stood behind her desk. Her shoulder-length, coffee-colored hair stuck out from a messy bun. A single diamond earring glittered in her left ear, and her usual wide grin had been replaced by a tight, weary expression. If she hadn't been wearing her official unit jacket, I'd have thought she'd come in drunk.

"Oh, hey, Megan. I didn't know you'd be coming in today." She frowned. "What *are* you doing here?"

"I came in to see if there were any extras. Tami said you were looking for me. Have you gotten my results from the CCRN class yet?"

Her mouth bobbed up and down for a second before she motioned to a chair. "Oh, uh, no. I haven't heard back yet. Have a seat. I'm glad you stopped by. I need to speak with you."

My backpack fell to the floor with a thud as I lowered myself into an old chair. "Looking good," I said with a little smile, surveying her haggard expression.

Her lips twitched. "I could say the same about you."

"You need coffee."

"More like an espresso drip."

"Seriously, Karen. Are you—"

She waved me off. "Fine. I'm fine. Just a bit tired."

Paperwork lay scattered across her desktop. Minutes from a meeting. Immunization records. Next month's schedule. Licensure renewals highlighted in red, the word *URGENT* screaming across the top. Karen steepled her hands in front of her and drew in a deep breath. My stomach knotted like an old necklace.

I sat back. "This can't be good."

"As you know, the hospital is struggling financially and has been for a while. To stay ahead of The Game, our CEO is asking every unit to cut back." Her eyes fluttered closed, and her shoulders slumped. "On staff."

The light in her office clouded. My mouth worked like a fish for ten seconds before any words came out.

"Cut back?"

"We have to downsize by one full-time nurse." She sucked in a deep breath through her teeth. Her voice had become a monotone. "Unfortunately, that's you."

My mind whirled. I had no seniority at West End. Before hiring on last year, I'd been at another hospital in a Pediatric ICU. For the past six years, I'd moved units often so I could gain more experience in preparation for flight nursing.

My blood iced in my veins.

"Me?" I whispered.

"I know it's unexpected. An ironic twist of fate to lose one of our best nurses because of a numbers game. Unfortunately, I have no way around it." She shuffled through a stack of papers. "I've tried to negotiate. I've looked for someone else to let go, but I don't have enough documentation of error."

She pressed her fingertips to her forehead. A long silence filled the vacuum. The marrow of my bones had been sucked away. Not only would I lose my job but possibly my perfectly structured career. My chance of becoming a flight-nurse teetered on thin ice.

Karen's heavy exhale drew me out of my winnowing thoughts. She pinched the bridge of her nose between her thumb and forefinger.

"Megan, I wish I could tell you how sorry I am."

"The flight team," I said, stuttering. "I'm so close! I've done every certification class. There's a new opening on the flight team in just a few months. Blake accepted my application two weeks ago."

"Maybe Blake can work magic that I can't. Trust me, Megan." She put a hand over her face. "I've tried everything."

My fervor died. This cutback would hurt more than just me. The entire floor would suffer, including Karen.

"It's not your fault." I swallowed. "I can see that you've tried, and that means a lot."

"One of my friends, Jodie Renner, is a nurse recruiter for EveryHealth Corporation. I'm going to send your name her way. She'll get you a job." Karen's voice softened. "Just ... not at West End."

The words settled in my mind, trailing into a numb haze.

Not at West End.

Karen set her shoulders. "The severance package is minimal. Four weeks paid. Unfortunately, I need you to clean out your locker and hand over your badge before you leave. I'm sorry, Megan, but we won't be staffing you anymore."

I drifted into a numb stupor while Karen moved into the details about severance pay and insurance benefits through the summer.

All effective immediately.

2

COME HOME

The moment I stepped into the parking garage, I whipped out my phone, flipped through my contacts, and pressed Blake's name. Blake, Flight Team Director, could fix this.

He had to.

Without my badge bouncing on my chest with every step, I felt naked. Shock propelled me through the parking garage on autopilot. The ringing stopped, and a familiar, deep voice answered.

"This is Blake."

"Blake! It's Megan. You'll never believe what just happened."

"NSYNC is going on tour again?"

I stopped. "Seriously? That's your guess?"

"Don't judge me."

"Karen just laid me off."

Silence.

"Blake? You there?"

"She did *what*?"

I ran through the conversation in a maniacal ramble, adding bits here and there as I remembered them, like a kindergartener using glue and paper for the first time. My fingers ached from squeezing the phone.

"Please tell me you can fix this. Please."

"Meg ... I don't know."

"Randy's still retiring next month, right? Which means there'll be an open slot. I can still apply even if I'm not employed by West End." I pressed the phone to my ear until it crackled. "Right?"

"First of all, I need you to take a deep breath."

"I'm calm!" I snapped.

"Take it, Megan."

Balking at his commanding tone, I obeyed. "Okay," I said through gritted teeth. "I'm calm now."

"The hospital owns the flight team, which means they'll use internal hires first."

"Can you hire outsiders?"

His long pause felt like a death gong. "Not if I have qualified internal applicants."

"Do you?"

"Several. I'm sorry, Meg. I can't hire you."

Every challenging class, every night shift, every lost patient, and every sacrifice funneled into a finite, articulated point. The flight team. All of it turned to stone in my body, weighing me down to the very core of the earth. I wanted to sink into it and disappear. To forget Nathan. Karen. To erase the last twenty-four hours and start over again. How could I lose so much in so little time?

Tears clouded my eyes. "I see," I whispered.

"I can make some calls. Look around. But we have three other candidates."

"Thanks." I cleared my throat. "I appreciate your honesty. Let me know if you hear of any other opportunities, will you?"

"No problem, Meg. I'm really so sorry."

A hot and stinging tear slipped down my cheek. I wiped it away with the back of my hand.

"Yeah. Me too."

What Do I Do Now?

- *Forrest Gump this place and never stop running.*
- *Buy more of those things that taste salty.*
- *Try to—*
- *~~Call Lexie and then—~~*
- *~~Call the twins.~~*
- *~~Call Mom.~~*
- *Food?*
- *Live out of a van?*
- *Stop staring at the dirt mark on the wall.*

MY PHONE RANG FAR TOO EARLY the next morning.

The annoying bell reverberated through my head in thick, heavy waves. Why was my alarm on? I didn't work until Saturday. Nathan sometimes called early to check my schedule. The ringing stopped. In the silence, lucidity brushed the dust of my fractured sleep away. No work. No Nathan. No flight team.

I sank back into my pillows and tried to melt into the mattress. My head throbbed, and my eyes burned like hot sandpaper. The black screen of my laptop stared at me with damning judgment. It had run out of battery while I was looking for another job. Nothing that would get me back on track for flight nursing had come up within two hundred miles. In desperation, I'd even applied to a travel-nurse company before the computer shut off.

"Nursing shortage my—"

The phone rang again. With a growl, I scrambled toward it. Video call with my brother Mark. Fantastic. The last thing I needed was the twins prying into my issues. In true brotherly fashion, they always wanted to fix everything.

A couple blind jabs later, I hit the green circle.

"'Lo?"

"Little blister, why do you hate us?" Mark asked, his nose wrinkling. "And showering, apparently."

I rolled onto my back with a yawn.

"I always look this way."

The picture juggled until JJ's high cheekbones and bemused hazel eyes appeared. For being twins, they looked nothing alike. JJ wore his chocolate-brown hair in a man bun, while Mark kept his light brown hair short and messy.

"Hey, Megara," JJ said. "Where've you been? I've been married twice and had five kids since you last called."

"I talked to you last week. Did you get my check for Adventura?"

"Yes, sugar mama. Many thanks. We appreciate the investment. Turns out running a summer camp takes a lot of money. You look like hell, by the way."

"Thanks."

"Anytime."

Last fall, Mark found an abandoned summer camp for sale in the Rocky Mountains. Within a week, he sweet-talked a handful of investors and bought it. Upgrades on Adventura Boys Camp had been ongoing for months now in preparation for its inaugural week in June.

Mark appeared on the screen again. I leaned against the headboard. "I didn't know you had internet at camp," I said, brow furrowed.

"We're at the Frolicking Moose Coffee Shop in Pineville bumming off theirs. We have decent cell reception in some spots but no internet. Speaking of camp, Adventura is why we called."

A moment of panic clutched my stomach. I hadn't logged into my checking account for a few days. "The check didn't bounce, did it?"

"No, and thanks for that, by the way. That will help a lot. Listen, our chef just bailed. Some health issues popped up out of nowhere, and he can't work for us."

"Doesn't Adventura open in a week?"

"Don't remind me."

"That's too bad. But what does that have to do with me?"

"Want it?"

I paused. "Uh … want what?"

"Two brothers in an eternal debt of gratitude and subject to your every whim. Or, in other words, the job as chef at Adventura Boys Camp."

"You're kidding."

Mark pressed his lips together. "Nope."

"You can't be serious."

"But I am."

"Mark, I don't know anything about cooking for teenagers. Or strangers. Or more than three people. Plus, everything I fix is healthy, and you hate healthy."

I thought of dinner the previous night and pushed the empty carton of ice cream onto a pile of unopened bills with my toe. Mostly healthy, anyway.

"I don't hate healthy in theory, just in taste," he said. "Besides, you'd only cook for the staff. Twenty people max on the weekends. Ten during the week. The kids cook for themselves in their campsites. Teaches them how to be men and all that."

JJ came on the screen. "The benefits of the job are unbelievable, Meg. No insurance. No paycheck. No air conditioning. The only guarantee is that you'll be so annoyed by the heat in the kitchen that you'll shave your head and save money on hair products."

Mark rubbed the back of his neck. "We're over budget with repairs and underpaying the rest of our staff. Our previous cook was doing it for free as a favor, so we'd kind of need you to do the same."

My brow grew heavy over my eyes. "So not only do you want me to leave for a month—"

"Two and a half months, actually. Last week of camp ends August 4th."

"—but you want me to do it for free?"

Both of them grinned, as if there were something amusing about their desperation.

"Yep."

Would I want to move back to the mountains, chain myself to a kitchen, and slave away in front of a stove for hours? Maybe a little. Being with the twins would be worth far more pain. Cooking for a handful of people couldn't be that hard, anyway. It wasn't like West End needed me anymore.

Mark brought the phone close to his face. Flecks of gold filled his hazel eyes. "If you say no, you basically hate fun."

"Define fun," I said.

"Moose. Dirt. Bugs the size of your face." Mark waved his hand in front of him. "The smell of campfire as your own natural musk. There's a ghost bear that we hear but never see. So, that's safe. Besides, I wouldn't even make you sign a contract. That's how much I trust you, blister."

"And you know how much he loves contracts, Meg. He made me sign one, and I'm part-owner."

"You make it sound so irresistible," I said.

"Just try not to fly in tonight. I'll even promise you JJ's firstborn," Mark said.

"JJ has no plans to reproduce."

"She's not wrong," JJ said.

"Adventura is amazing, Meg." Mark leaned toward the phone. "It's freedom. It's mountains. It's ... it's home, all right? You have to come home. We miss you."

His impassioned plea tugged at my heart. It had been too long since I'd climbed a mountain. Smelled the forest. Drunk from a stream. The ghosts of IV machines and heart monitors beeped in my mind, and I couldn't decide if I'd miss them. Could I afford to leave for two months? Probably not. Dating Nathan had taken a toll on my credit card. The abysmal job offerings from last night ran back through my mind.

What else would occupy my time for two months if not twelve-hour shifts in a hospital?

"Stay home, Meg." JJ leaned back, stacking his hands behind his head with a yawn. "Then Mom can cook, and we'll be those cool thirty-year-olds who hang out with their parents all summer."

I perked up. "Yeah! What about Mom? She'd be great."

A shadow passed over Mark's face. "Mom has her own stuff going on this summer. And we wanted to hang out with you again. Anyway, it was worth a shot. No worries, sis. We get it. You hate us."

"Not true. Can I ... can I just think about it?"

"Of course. Call us back in—" He checked his watch. "—twelve hours. If you can't, we have to find someone else."

Once we ended the call, I sank back into the covers and stared at the streams of sunlight flooding through the window and spilling onto the floor. Living in the mountains again sounded like a dream. But my thoughts drifted over the reasons I shouldn't leave for two months. Money, for one. Job progression, for another. My friends, for a third.

My mind went blank after that.

With a sigh, I shoved off the covers and headed for the shower. Twelve hours and counting.

Later that night, I sat on the floor with my back against the couch. An old rerun of *Home Improvement* played in the background while the paper foliage of my finances fanned around me. Plumbers. Mortgage. Car payment. It added up to an ugly arithmetic.

Traveler's Credit Card.

Minimum Balance Due: $50.91.

The full balance lingered at just over $2,000, a sum I had no hope of paying without a job. I sucked in a breath with a hiss. Why had I given the twins so much money to invest in Adventura? Had I really needed to spend two hundred dollars on a cocktail dress for Nathan's gala? The four weeks' severance would cover my mortgage and car payment for June but not much more. Paying off the credit card would have to wait.

At 18% interest.

I tilted my head back, resting it on the couch. I'd never been in debt before. Correction: I'd never been jobless, single, *and* in debt before. I reached for my phone to text Mark.

Sorry, bro. Finances don't add up.

A knock at my front door startled me just as my thumb hovered over the *send* button. I tossed it aside to send later, shoved my papers and laptop under the couch, and hopped to my feet. Until I decided what direction my life would take, discretion was key. The Health and Happiness Society didn't need to know my life was in shambles. Eventually, I'd get around to telling them about my breakup, job loss, and horrific financial situation.

Just ... not yet.

Outside, four familiar voices jumbled together.

"No, Lexie, we didn't order an extra egg roll."

"No lecture on MSG, Bitsy?"

"One meal with MSG isn't going to kill us."

"Repeated exposure causes cancer."

"Drink lemon water. It flushes it out. You'll be fine."

When I threw open the door, the rest of the Health and Happiness Society beamed at the same time. "Megan!" they cried in unison. I widened the door, beckoning them in with a smile and a wave.

"Come on in, ladies."

Lexie held up two brown bags. "We brought Chinese food! The gods of takeout have smiled on us: Bitsy approved."

"Only for broccoli beef," Bitsy said, wagging a finger. "The rest are just—"

Lexie rolled her eyes, darting past me like an arrow. "Cooked MSG popsicles. We know."

Except for Little Debbie snacks, nothing made Lexie happier than Chinese food. Well, maybe Chipotle. Her trailing blonde hair spilled in strands of sunshine from a high ponytail as she whipped by. The gym had brought us together when she started working out for the first time. In the year and a half since, she had slenderized and toned down, finding an oval face and a sturdy pair of shoulders.

Rachelle, Lexie's childhood best friend, slipped by me with a wink. The heady scent of an alluring perfume hovered in her wake. My eyes darted from her leather jacket to the rip that raced up the back of her fishnet tights. She'd lost over seventy-five pounds since she joined the Health and Happiness Society last fall.

"I brought the ice cream you texted me about," she whispered. "Bitsy doesn't know yet, but it's in my purse. I'll slip it into your freezer."

I gave her a discreet thumbs-up. Rachelle always had my back.

Bitsy and Mira spilled in last. Bitsy, a single mom of two young girls, wore creamy gray slacks and a button-up shirt. She slipped out of a modest pair of pumps with a happy sigh.

"Thanks for having us this week, Megan," she said.

"Anytime."

"Hullo, Megan, my dear." Mira flapped a chubby hand in front of her face. "Oh, it feels good in here. It's starting to get hot outside. I hate summer."

Her fluffy hair ballooned into a halo in the evening humidity, but it was her makeup that caught my eye. Her bright orange eye shadow—a near-perfect match for her loose dress—looked like a construction zone sign. I followed them into the living room, where Tim Allen grunted from the TV.

Bitsy's gaze narrowed on me as I grabbed the remote and shut the TV off. "You all right? You seem ... off."

I smiled. "Fine."

Lexie put her hands on her hips. "Your eyes are swollen."

Rachelle pointed to my feet. "She's wearing the yellow socks."

"And you have reruns of *Home Improvement* on TV," Mira said.

"Oh, no," Lexie whispered, one hand over her mouth. "This is your breakup routine. Did Nathan … did he…"

I scoffed. "I don't have a breakup routine."

They stared at me. In the past year, I'd gone through two other breakups with them at my side. My shoulders slumped. Okay. I probably had a breakup routine.

So much for discretion.

"Fine," I muttered. "Nathan broke up with me."

Lexie shoved me onto the couch.

"Spill."

Lexie and Bitsy passed around cartons and chopsticks while I explained. When I finished, Mira patted my hand, and Rachelle stabbed a chopstick into a carton of beef. "Good riddance, loser," Rachelle said.

Lexie reached over and hugged me. I absorbed it like a dry sponge, choking back tears.

"Thanks, Lex," I whispered.

Bitsy straightened. "We're on call for girlmergencies anytime. Just don't think you'll always get Chinese food with it. Mira, would you like to start the meeting? Please share your good news. We'll go around the circle."

Mira blushed as she mentioned missing two workouts because of dates with Pat, Lexie's boss and a local pub owner. Rachelle had landed a lucrative, full-time summer job that would make her *thousands of dollars just for watching an old man sleep and occasionally handing him his meds*, and Bitsy had found an investor for her housekeeping business.

"He wants to begin this month." Bitsy leaned back, her eyes alight. "I'm interviewing interior decorators next week so we can get started. It's going to be very busy this summer."

Lexie cleared her throat, casting a long glance at me out of the corner of her eye. "Well." She cleared her throat. "I have … uh … some news."

"You're pregnant!" Rachelle said.

Lexie paled. "No! Are you kidding? We haven't even … I mean, that's not … don't just drop that out there." She cleared her throat. "Bradley and I went ring shopping last week."

My heart bucked. I tightened my grip on my rice carton. Bitsy gasped.

Mira clapped, the loose flaps of skin on her arms wriggling. Lexie and Bradley had been long-distance dating for almost a year, but she'd never mentioned *marrying* him.

"What?" Rachelle screeched. "When? Where?"

"Tell us everything," Bitsy said.

A blush illuminated Lexie's fair cheeks. She bit her bottom lip, averting her eyes. "Well, we didn't buy anything. Just looked. I have chubby fingers! I wanted to try on a ring or two just in case." She rubbed her ring finger with her right hand. "He'll decide which one to buy, and he promised it would be a surprise. It could be any day now."

Married? But ... where did this come from? When did they start talking about such a serious commitment? Nathan's words played back through my head like a ticker tape, tightening my throat.

We just didn't have that it factor.

We just didn't have that it factor.

We just didn't have that it factor.

"He also wants me to meet his family," Lexie said, drawing me out of my thoughts. "I'm so scared I could pee. What if they don't like me?"

Underneath my haze of disbelief, a prickle warned me that Bitsy had locked in on my reaction. Sure enough, when I glanced over at her, she was staring me down with a mixture of concern and question. I swallowed and pasted on a dazzling smile.

"Congratulations, Lex," I said, wrapping her in a hug. "You and Bradley will make the cutest babies. I'm so happy for you."

Inside, I shriveled away.

The conversation rolled on. Lexie gushed about wedding plans while I picked at my rice. No matter what level of happiness I felt on Lexie's behalf, my chest ached. Lexie—in her first and very successful relationship—would get married and move away. Just like Dana.

And Elizabeth.

And Jodie.

As my best friends graduated to marriage, I'd clung to my career. Nursing had never let me down. Until it did. I couldn't even hold onto a boyfriend for more than a few months lately.

What is keeping me here? I thought, managing a half-hearted laugh at something Rachelle said. No job. No relationship. A best friend who would slowly slip away into her new life without me. Tears welled up in my eyes, but I blinked them back.

Nothing. Nothing is keeping me here.

With my phone hidden behind my knees, I started a new text to both JJ and Mark. Typing out the two words settled the boiling pain in my chest.

I'm in.

A flood of relief consumed me. The mountains. Lifting with Mom between meals. Mark and JJ and Dad setting marshmallows on fire. Repairing my broken heart by hiking every morning.

Mom and I had always been able to talk for hours—I could tell her everything without shame. Dad and I would go to Rudy's Diner for our favorite hamburgers. How much work could cooking for a handful of guys be, anyway? This would be a veritable two-month vacation in the mountains.

My phone buzzed. Mark.

You're a wise little blister. We can't wait to see you.

3

YOUR NEW KINGDOM

One week later.

The quiet rocking of the plane to Jackson City had lulled me into a doze. I jerked awake at the turbulence of the landing, my forehead pressed against the chilly, plastic windowpane. I'd stayed up half the night packing, cleaning, and reassuring Lexie that a bear wouldn't eat me. Considering I'd originally told her about the trip via text message because I was too much of a coward to say it to her face, she'd handled the announcement with grace. And fifty replies.

Dry air welcomed me into the terminal with a gentle embrace, so unlike the walls of humidity in the Midwest. Outside, mountains pierced the sky with jagged teeth of snow and granite. I tossed my backpack over my shoulder and shuffled through the airport, yawning.

First order of business once I arrived at Adventura: take a nap.

Running late, Mark said in a text.

Where are you?

Chasing tornados.

Of course.

We'll be there soon. Ish.

I eyed an empty bank of chairs. Would it be weird to nap in the middle of the airport? Deciding that Mark would tie me to the chair if he caught me, I moved on to baggage claim.

A crowd of people clumped around a wheezy carousel as it belched duffel bags. Locating my ratty suitcase a few steps away, I grabbed the handle to wrench it free, but the wheel caught. My wrist twisted as the bag tumbled to the ground. The zipper split with a *crack*.

Clothes spewed out like a cotton volcano.

"You've got to be kidding me," I muttered, scrabbling after a pair of polka-dot underwear and a runaway tampon. A teenager guffawed while I seized a purple bra. Honestly. Of all the bras to lose in the airport...

"Airports are the worst place to lose your underwear," said a man in a worn baseball hat. He set my hiking boots next to me with an amused twinkle in his eye. "Looks like your boots are getting a head start on you."

"Uh, yeah ... they've always had a mind of their own."

His shocking blue-gray eyes reminded me of a faded pair of jeans. His lip twitched, deepening a dimple in his right cheek. He hesitated, then reached past several pairs of underwear for a stray hoodie. Cheeks burning, I swept all the underwear into my arms and punched them into the corner of the suitcase.

Once we finished re-packing my bag, he stretched out a hand. I hesitated, looking from his callused palms back to his shadowed face, then accepted. He pulled me to my feet.

"Thanks for the help." I gestured to the bag. And for not embarrassing me over the colors of my underwear.

He shrugged it off, adjusting a backpack strap on his shoulder. My hand fell back to my side, tingling.

"I'm Justin," he said.

"Megan."

"Megan?" He tilted his head.

"Yeah. Why?"

His dimple deepened again. I'd been wrong. His eyes weren't denim but thunderstorm gray. Layers of amusement colored his tone. "Good to officially meet you."

A familiar cry jerked me back to reality.

"Yoo-hoo! Littlest blister! Over here!"

Two familiar oafs strode into baggage claim holding up signs that said,

THAT'S MY SISTER. THE ONE WITH THE FACE and *THE BLISTER HAS RETURNED.* A knee-high dog with gleaming black fur trotted next to them.

"Oh, Megan," Mark sang. "It's so good to see you."

I backed away two steps, palm raised.

"Don't you—"

He charged, wrapped his thick arms around my shoulders, and yanked me off my feet with his violent love. My scalp burned under a brotherly knuckle rub.

"Let me go!"

"Never!"

I nipped the fleshy part of his arm with my fingertips. He leaped back with a howl, releasing me.

"No fatty pinching!"

"Wimp."

Mark set his hands on his hips, studying me with a burgeoning grin. "In love and war, I suppose. It's good to see you, blister."

"It's always war with you, Mark."

He hauled me into a bear hug with a growl.

"You're a rotten brother," I said into his shoulder, but I squeezed him tight. Unlike JJ, who had a lean runner's body and muscular calves that belonged in a magazine, Mark had the meaty shoulders and legs of a weightlifter. They both loomed above me at six feet tall.

JJ jerked me away and tucked me into his arms.

"Took you long enough to return," he muttered. His chocolate-brown hair coiled in a bun at the back of his head. A scruffy beard had filled out his face, hiding a strong jaw and cheekbones that made most girls swoon. JJ knew his power.

I pulled away, flicking his bear-claw necklace.

"Real classy. Fake?"

JJ squeezed my shoulder. "Remind me to tell you the story. It involves a leprechaun, a sage old Native American man who I later find out is a ghost, and me wrestling a bear."

I laughed. "Naturally."

Mark grabbed my backpack and slung it over his shoulder, then shoved a brown paper bag into my chest. "You hungry? We already bought lunch.

That's why we were late. We got you tots. 'Cause you'll always be our little tater."

"And there's Justus Aurelius, the gladiator," JJ said, embracing the stranger who had helped me repack my clothes. "Your canine missed you, brother."

My mouth dropped.

Justin knew my brothers?

I elbowed Mark in the side. "You know that guy?" I asked while JJ and *Justus Aurelius* thumped each other on the back. Mark grabbed my bag, glancing over his shoulder as he headed toward the exit.

"Who? Justin?"

"Yeah."

He scoffed. "Of course we know him, Meg. The man is a freaking gladiator. Try not to fall in love with him, all right? He's part-owner of Adventura. And that would, quite frankly, just get weird."

~

My hopes of a nap dwindled with surprising speed.

JJ and Justin spoke quietly in the backseat the whole hour-long ride to Adventura. Snippets of their conversation drifted through my mind. *Grandpa* and *assets* and *lawyers*. I stayed in the front with Mark, grateful for a chance to compose myself after the embarrassment at the airport.

My purple bra. I pressed my forehead against the windowpane. *Polka-dot underwear. Seriously.*

Mark narrated a tour of Adventura as we drove through it, skimming past the glittering blue lake and thousands of lodgepole pines.

"Cell reception is best at the lodge and the main office. None at the ranges, but we'll use radios to communicate. Sorry, blister, but you'll have to explore it on your own time," he said as we bounced down a dirt road. "We have work to do."

Adventura sat at the base of two mountain canyons. The archery and rifle ranges occupied the northern area, the lake filled the west, the parking lot and main office lay at the southern edge, and campsites scattered the eastern side. A lodge and the trading post stood right in the middle.

When I stepped out of Mark's truck, the bracing scent of wildflowers filled my lungs. Craggy peaks blocked most of the sky, casting long, cool shadows. In the distance, a creek bubbled.

"Sweet chariot, Mark." I reached for my backpack when Mark dropped the tailgate. Deep, rusted tire rims blended with the fading marmalade of the chipped paint. Inside, a woven mat partially covered a frisbee-sized hole in the middle seat.

"It gets me all the ladies."

"Where'd you get it?"

"Bought it from a guy in Jackson City for a hundred bucks. It'll withstand the zombie invasion, little blister. Tease me now, but you'll be sorry when the zombies come."

The left bumper dropped with a groan.

"You better pray for slow zombies." I slung my backpack over my shoulder. JJ retrieved my broken suitcase and headed toward a one-room cabin off to the right. Justin faded into the trees, calling for his dog with a punctuated, three-note whistle.

Mark kicked the bumper back up.

"C'mon," he said. "I'll show you your luxurious private condo. Pets allowed. Hope you like squirrels."

Dust billowed beneath my backpack when I dropped it in the middle of the musty wooden structure. Cobwebs swept out from the rustic logs in gossamer curtains. Dead bugs overflowed from the windowsills. No cot. No shelves. No water source. Nothing but dusty air and rotting wood.

"We can move you to a less ornate space if you'd like," JJ said.

"It's..."

Mark ducked around a cobweb. "Impressive?"

"Clean?" JJ grinned.

"Dry," I said.

JJ eyed a beam of sunlight streaming through a fist-sized hole in the ceiling. "For now."

"Just wait till you see the kitchen," Mark muttered. "Let's go check it out. JJ will get you a sleeping bag. I think we have a cot around here somewhere. The gladiator will know."

JJ made a sign of the cross. "May you survive without disease or maiming. I'll wait here."

"Scared?" I asked.

He smirked. "You should be, too."

With JJ's warning ringing in my ears, I followed Mark. He gestured to the left, where a cabin hid behind tree boughs.

"That's Justin's cabin."

His roof sloped more steeply than mine, and white lines of insulation puffed out from between the hefty logs like a gingerbread house. A tangled lump of saplings separated us, joined by a ribbon-like footpath cutting between the trees. I turned away, my cheeks warm.

Not far from my cabin, a sprawling, rectangular building with a crooked *Lodge* sign sat at the edge of a meadow. Its covered front porch faced away from my cabin. Mark led me through the loose screen door at the back.

"This is your new kingdom, blister."

One of four fluorescent tubes flickered to life at the flip of the light switch, casting an anemic glow on the cramped room. I stopped in the doorway, bracing myself. My eyes widened.

"Oh."

The kitchen had an open, mildewed fridge, two sinks that shared a hanging spigot, and a restaurant-sized grill. An island counter occupied the middle of the room, leaving room for one person to walk around. The bottoms had fallen out of two cupboards along the wall. Cobwebs lined the rafters like a layer of thick frosting. Next to the grill, two holes smaller than my fist had been eaten into the wall at the floor seam.

"What do you think?" he asked.

I swallowed, nudging the fridge door closed. It swung open again. "Is ... this it?"

"Uh-huh."

"It's ... ah ... yep."

He kicked aside the carcass of a beetle. "The potential has rendered you speechless, I see. I will concede that it needs some cleaning."

"More like the full force of a thousand scrubbing bubbles."

"We have two gallons of Windex."

"Should be enough for the windows..."

"Five containers of bleach?"

"That'll cover the floor," I murmured, unable to decipher whether the floor in question was tile or dirt.

Mark patted me on the back. "You got this, blister. It's why we called you. We needed the best."

"Cleaning *is* my superpower," I said.

"I thought it was being annoying."

"I'm multifaceted."

He grinned, smacking me on the back again.

"Ah, blister. It's been boring without you."

Despite my love of tackling a dirty surface and exposing the gleam beneath, I'd need a fairy-godmother-sized miracle. I eyed the foggy windowpanes over the sink with growing reservations.

"Where have you been cooking during renovations?" I asked.

He snorted. "Real men microwave. And eat a lot of cold cereal in the office. This fridge isn't working yet. I have a repair guy coming in this weekend. Oh, there's a pantry." He pointed to a thin door opposite us. "Don't go in there until you have some kind of mask, though."

"Ha. Right."

His expression didn't falter. "Not kidding."

"You're serious?"

"I never kid about noxious mold."

He ran his palm over the smooth surface of the grill. Dust bunnies gathered on his fingertips, and he flicked them away. "Also, we're not sure if the grill works. And before you go crazy on loaves of homemade bread, a squirrel may be living in one of the two ovens, so do a critter check first."

He strode through a swinging door that led into the rest of the lodge. I stared, blinking. Wait. Did he say *homemade bread*? I followed, eager to escape the stinky confines of my new office.

"Wait a second. No one said anything about homemade brea—"

I stopped in a cavernous room with an open ceiling and smooth, cement floor. Half a dozen tables with benches crowded one side. A blackened, empty fireplace filled the wall on the opposite end. The rampant dust lent it an old-world charm. At least I had someplace cool to escape. That kitchen would broil like the furnaces of hell come July.

"The staff will eat and meet here." Mark stood in the middle of the room, his lips pursed as he stared into the rafters. The gauzy strands of a spider web floated by, and the smell of pine drifted into the room.

"Keeping this place clean will also be my responsibility?" I trailed a finger along a dusty windowsill.

He clicked his tongue as he pointed at me. "Nailed it. We'll have campers in here for crafts on Wednesdays. But otherwise, you own it."

"Great."

He jammed his hands into his front pockets, his wide shoulders angular in his loose t-shirt. His obvious adoration for such a helpless place reminded me of an overly proud papa that wanted to show the world his wrinkled, squalling new baby.

"So," he drawled. "What do you think of Adventura so far?"

A single sentence couldn't contain my thoughts. They'd clearly worked hard to bring Adventura up to date. Fresh roofs on the staff cabins. A brand new dock at the waterfront. The camp pulsed with its own current of life, as if the trees anticipated the bustle of the coming weeks. I felt as if I'd been taken from real life and set on a new planet. One that stirred my blood with the song of the mountains.

"I think it's ... wonderful," I said.

His eyebrows shot up. "Really?"

I grinned. "Yeah. I mean, the kitchen is horrific. We'll probably die of some incurable disease before it's cleaned. But the rest of Adventura is great. You've worked hard, Mark. I'm really proud of you."

"Yeah?"

"Yeah." I nodded, returning his enthusiastic smile. "This is amazing."

He slapped both hands on my shoulders and spun me around, steering me back to the kitchen. The puff of his chest gave him away.

"All right. Cheesy time is over. Get your grubby little hands on a bottle of bleach. I'm not paying you the big bucks to stand around and talk about how much you love me, am I?"

~

Kitchen Supplies and Shopping List

- *Biohazard signs*
- *Sponges the size of my face*
- *A gallon of hydrochloric acid*

- *Drywall*
- *Spider bombs*
- *Shoe inserts for Mark's stinky feet*
- *Dog treats to bribe Atticus*
- *A hungry, vicious cat*
- *Gas masks*

THAT EVENING, I stood in the middle of my cabin and stared at a sleeping bag and foam pad from JJ. With a pair of sweats and a hoodie, it would be warm enough for tonight.

"Sleeping on the floor it is," I said. Granted, I hadn't expected a resort or maid service. Or squirrels as roommates.

A lantern hanging from the rafters shed yellow light onto the wooden floor, which I'd swept clean twice already. Somehow, pine needles littered the floor again. I didn't dare unpack my suitcase—where would I put everything? I thought about walking to the office, where Mark and JJ slept in the attic, but decided against it. My head throbbed. I just wanted to sleep, even on the ground.

I eyed my extra hoodies. They'd make a decent pair of drapes for the night, which would keep out some of the cold. I'd stuff a shirt full of clothes to use as a pillow...

A knock on the screen door startled me.

"Just me," Justin called through the screen. "I have a few things for you."

I stepped back. "Oh, sure. Come on in."

His beautiful dog slipped in ahead of him, black coat gleaming in the light. Justin propped open the door, dragging something metal behind him. My eyes widened, and I crossed my arms over my chest in horror. I'd already taken off my bra! A pair of JJ's old high school wrestling sweats—threadbare and baggy—hung off my hips. With a messy braid and no makeup, I'd likely stun Justin with my dazzling au-natural appearance.

For sure.

Then again ... what did it matter? He'd already seen my underwear.

A metal contraption slid into the middle of the room, squeaking in protest. "I brought you a cot." He smiled, pressing the folded ends into a waist-high bed, his bronzed muscles flexing with each movement. I swallowed, forcing my gaze back to the rusty cot before he caught me ogling.

"That will be far more comfortable than the floor. Thank you so much."

He straightened, assessing the bare windows and open hole in the ceiling. "These cabins aren't exactly built for luxury."

"Really? I hadn't noticed."

He chuckled, one finger held up. "Just a second. There are a few more things."

He disappeared back outside, reappearing seconds later with a long, round dowel, a hammer, and eight nails between his teeth.

"Makeshift closet," he said around the nails. A minute later, he'd nailed the dowel across the south back corner, creating a bar for me to hang my clothes. He stepped back, surveyed it, and nodded in satisfaction.

"I have some extra hangers in my cabin," he said, stepping to the middle of the wall and grabbing another nail. He drove the last four nails into the wood at eye level, each one a foot apart. "Some extra pegs for towels and stuff. Without cupboards, these will come in handy. I'll come back tomorrow and make you a shelf by the windows."

"Oh, wow. Thanks! You've got this wilderness living down, huh?"

"I'm a regular Tarzan."

"I can't wait to see you talk to the animals then." I eyed the open windows. "You wouldn't be hiding any extra drapes in your loincloth, would you, Tarzan?"

He laughed. "No, but I do know where some old pillowcases are hanging out. Want me to grab them?"

"Oh, I don't mind doing it. Where are they?"

He waved it off. "I'll be right back. Mind if Atticus stays?" He gestured to the dog. I raised an eyebrow.

"Atticus, huh? Are you a loyal fan of *To Kill a Mockingbird*?"

A little blush misted the apples of his cheeks. "Harper Lee and I are basically best friends."

I laughed. "Yes, please leave him. I love dogs."

Once he departed, I reached down to pet Atticus while staring at the modifications. The room already seemed smaller without Justin in it. Shaking my head, I thrust the cot against the far wall and tossed the pad and sleeping bag on top. The silky material slid through my fingertips like cool water. Atticus stared at me from the floor, his head cocked to one side. I nodded to the cot.

"Wanna?"

With a graceful leap, he jumped on top, circled the sleeping bag, and sprawled out, tail twitching. I ran a hand through his thick, smooth fur and rubbed his ears. He groaned and leaned into it.

"You're a handsome devil."

By the time Justin returned, I'd started to unpack, flinging a jacket, a towel, my hiking boots, and my tennis shoes on the nails in the wall. He entered with two pillowcases draped over his shoulder and a handful of wire hangers he set on my new closet dowel.

"Feels like home already," he said.

"I think I'll be a modern-day Laura Ingalls Wilder."

He chuckled, pulling two small nails from a pocket and wielding a hammer in his right hand as he strode to the first window.

"So," I asked, sitting on the cot next to Atticus. "How'd you find this handsome guy? He's gorgeous."

"I didn't. He found me."

His response hummed with an undercurrent that I didn't have the courage to wade into. If he'd wanted to tell me the story, he probably would have.

"And you met the twins in Costa Rica?"

A rueful grin found its way onto his attractive lips. He chuckled. "Yeah. A while ago, actually. Eight years, I think? Mark got into a bar fight on the beach, and JJ was a little too drunk himself to be of much use. I stepped in to help them out."

"Did you know them at the time?"

"Nope."

"You helped them out anyway?"

"Yep."

I wondered what he wasn't saying. Atticus rested his head on my thigh with a sigh. I buried my fingertips in his thick fur.

"And you became friends after that?" I asked.

"I guess they developed man crushes on me they can't get rid of."

I tilted my head back and laughed. He patted two nails into place at the top of the window, obscuring it with the white pillowcase, and moved to the next.

"Your brothers said you're a nurse," he said. "That's nice of you to leave your job to help them out here for free."

A worm of nervousness wriggled in my chest. I hadn't *exactly* told the twins the truth about losing my job when I'd mumbled something about extended leave and changes at the hospital. The pity on Bitsy's face when I'd finally confessed the truth to her hadn't motivated me toward total honesty with the twins.

"Uh, yeah."

Justin stepped back, studying the makeshift drape, and nodded in satisfaction. "That look okay?"

I straightened. "Fantastic. Thank you so much."

"No problem. Let me know if you need anything else." His eyes shot to the hole in the roof. "I put a piece of plastic over that earlier today and plan on fixing it before camp starts. Do you need anything else tonight?"

Nathan admitting how wrong he was for dumping me. A functioning job that pays well. And a real pillow.

"No," I said with a smile, rising to my feet. "This should be good, thank you. I'll sleep much better."

His gaze lingered on me for half a second before he gave me a thumbs-up. "All right. Well, have a good night, Meg. Atticus, come."

Atticus trotted away with Justin, fading into the night. Sighing, I sank onto the cot, and it creaked under my weight.

A new summer of being single, spending time with my brothers, and enjoying the mountains stretched out before me. Maybe it wouldn't be so bad here at Adventura. I could survive a summer without taking extra shifts or placing IVs. Running the kitchen would be easy. Besides, Mom was coming tomorrow. I could hash all of this out with her. Talk about Nate. My desperate job loss. As if I were a kid again, Mom would make it better.

I flopped back on my bag with a contented sigh.

Ah, mountain life.

4

SOMEHOW

Rain drummed on the kitchen ceiling early the next morning. A chill drove through my hoodie and deep into my bones. An old pair of rubber gloves squeaked against my hands as I stood in front of the pantry, bleach bottle at my side. I shoved my sleeves higher on my arms.

"All right, you moldy monster. Make my day."

The pantry door groaned open. I waited in vain for an attack of killer mold or a rancid blast of air. Instead, a beam of light illuminated a shredded bag of sugar on the floor. When I pulled a chain hanging in the middle of the pantry, nothing happened. I set a lantern on a shelf, spreading light through the cramped, L-shaped room. A tub of weevil-infested flour had fallen over, and tiny tracks ran through it. Generous piles of mouse droppings littered the floor.

"You are a brave woman, Megan Bailey, venturing into that pantry alone."

I whipped around. A wiry, lean woman with muscular legs stood just inside the kitchen, balancing a laundry basket filled with bottles of cleaning solution and new rolls of paper towels on her left hip. I grinned.

"I learned it from my mom."

"Sounds like a crazy woman."

"You should meet her."

A wide smile bloomed on Mom's face. Her warm caramel-brown hair shimmered with streaks of gray as it swung around her shoulder blades.

"Oh, Meg. It's so good to see you."

She set the laundry basket aside, closed the space between us, and enveloped me in her powerful arms. I pressed close, inhaling the tangy scent of home from her running jacket.

"I'm so relieved to see you," I breathed, pulling away. "I have so much to tell you. I don't even know where to start. And thank you for helping me clean. This kitchen is ... well ... you know."

"Anything for my favorite daughter."

"Only daughter," I quipped.

She winked. "Same thing."

She pressed a hand to my cheek with a warm smile, but it didn't quite reach her eyes. Lines ran like canyons from her eyes down her too-thin cheeks. Weariness clung to her like she hadn't slept in a week.

I put a hand on her arm.

"Mom, is everything all right?"

"All those lowlanders come up to the mountains in the summer and have heart attacks, so I've been pulling extras this week. You know how it is." She released a rueful sigh. "Flight nursing always keeps me on my toes."

"Did Dad come with you?"

"No." An edge of tension cut through her voice. "I ... think he's at work. Anyway, I brought you an extra cooler with ice. The fridge isn't working yet, is it?"

While she jabbered about rags and cleaning supplies, she flitted around the kitchen like a manic bee, never settling. She unloaded a bottle of window cleaner and degreaser onto the island, then set them next to the grill. With a tut, she transferred them to the windowsill.

"You sure everything's okay, Mom?" I asked, watching her search for a place for the garbage bags. She set them on the counter, then moved them to the grill and reached for something else in the basket. Then she thought better of it and went back for the bags.

"Fine! So, listen. I bought this vinegar-based cleaner—"

"Mom, wait. Before you unload everything, tell me what's going on. You're so jumpy you'd make coffee nervous."

"I'm just tired."

"But—"

Her shoulders tensed. "Nothing," she snapped. "Nothing is wrong. Just leave it alone, all right?"

I shrank back. She pressed a hand to her forehead and closed her eyes, leaning against the cluttered island. The muscles in her jaw tightened. Her shoulders stooped.

"I'm sorry." She met my worried gaze. "I shouldn't have snapped. I really am tired. Just ... leave it, Meg, for now. Please? I'm not ready to talk about it."

My heart leaped into my throat. *It.* So there *was* something going on.

"Okay. Sure. Let's talk about, uh, something else."

In silence, we fell into our separate duties. I shuffled back to the pantry, broom in hand, and swept up the sugar and flour. Mom stayed at the sink, staring out the window. Time stood still. Only the scratch of the broom on the floor broke the quiet. Just when I thought I couldn't stand another second, I felt a tentative touch on my back, light as a butterfly wing.

"Meg? I'm sorry."

I turned around to find her slumped against the wall, her head tilted back. Her eyes sparkled, as if she was holding back tears. I leaned on the broom handle.

"It's all right, Mom. Bad days come and go."

She sighed and rubbed the back of her neck. "It's not that. I just ... I'm frustrated with your father."

My throat tightened. "Is everything okay?'

"It's fine. Your father and I are fine. He's fine. I'm fine. It's all just *fine*. We've been *fine* ever since you guys left the house. Whenever I ask him, he says he's *fine*. He never asks me, so I just pretend that *I'm* fine. We just live in a big, damn circle of *fine*."

A rangy laugh bubbled out of her. She thrust away from the wall, snatched a brown bag from the basket, and yanked out a box of baking soda.

"You wouldn't believe how many years you can live on being *fine*. How many years you can tell yourself that everything will be *fine* even if you don't believe it. Or maybe you do believe it, because if you don't, you can't imagine what it would mean. So, it's easier to just be *fine* at any cost. Until, one day, it's not. And you realize you've been lying to yourself all those years."

I reached out and put my fingers over hers. She stilled. A hand rose to cover half her face. The mania in her motions calmed, and in its place settled a bone-deep weariness.

"Oh, Meg," she whispered. "I'm so sorry. I didn't mean to burden you. I'm just ... struggling."

"Mom, it's okay."

She fell against me with a little cry, like a terrified kitten. I wrapped my arms around her, paralyzed in shock. What could I even say? Mom and Dad having marriage problems?

"Are you fighting?" I finally managed, sounding hoarse. She pulled away, sniffling, using her knuckle to wipe away tears.

"Yes. We have been for a while. It's worse when we're together."

"Are you apart?"

"Not yet. Not officially, anyway."

My thoughts fractured into thousands of glittery shards. What did this mean? How had it happened? Did the twins know? How was Dad doing? The questions swung at me like wrecking balls. I'd come home hoping to cling to Mom, but for the first time in my life, she clung to me.

"Mom, it's okay. Look, we'll work this out. After all these years together, I'm sure you'll figure it out."

Mascara smeared under her right eye. She sniffled but didn't meet my eyes. Her deadpan voice didn't give me much hope. "I hope so, Meg. I really do."

"Do JJ and Mark know?"

"Mark knows. I don't think JJ does. Your father would be furious if he knew I told you. He doesn't want to worry anyone. Please don't tell your father or your brothers I told you. Please? It's very important to me that ... I don't know. I just ... I don't want everyone to know yet."

I winced. Dad furious with Mom? Sure, they'd had disagreements when I was growing up, like any married couple would. But Dad's long-fuse temper rarely manifested itself. I pushed aside all my worries over Lexie's impending marriage and my joblessness and the tower of bills. For now, I'd focus on Mom.

"I understand. I won't say anything."

"Thanks, Meg. Let's not talk about this anymore."

"Okay." I set my hands on my hips. "Let's clean this disaster up, eh? There's no therapy quite like manual labor. Or so my mother always told me."

A tremulous smile stole across her face, replacing the melancholy. She cleared her throat, resetting herself back to the can-conquer-all Mom I'd always known.

"That's my girl," she said, pressing a salty kiss onto my cheek. "Always works hard. Let's divide and conquer. This place needs a makeover."

Food List for Blister

- *Black Forest Cake. 'Nuff Said.*
- *Homemade bread*
- *Spaghetti—extra points for homemade sauce*
- *French toast*
- *LOTS OF EGGS.*
- *More. Black. Forest. Cake.*
- *Pepperoni Hot Pockets. NOT meatball. I'll fire you so fast...*
- *Raw veggies to a minimum. Like zero.*
- *Chicken pad thai.*
- *Chinese food.*
- *Greek Food. (Ten pounds of feta and a crap ton of falafel).*
- *Sione wants a pig to roast. Full pig. Face and everything.*
- *Constant Oreo supply.*

^ But seriously

- *BLACK FOREST CAKE.*

Note from JJ: Definitely buy fresh carrots and hummus if you can. Baby tomatoes are a win. I'll take celery, but it's not my favorite. Oh, and get natural PB.

THE CHILLY JUNE air breathed down my neck early the next morning, sending goosebumps down my arms. The heater in Mark's Zombie Mobile proved to be as consistent as my dating history. My breath curled out in front of me in light wisps as I rumbled down the mountain roads and pulled into Pineville.

Ahead of me, pink-and-white sunbursts opened behind the mountains, stretching with long arms into the sky. When I pulled in, the Pineville Market parking lot lay empty except for three other cars, one decorated with swirls of frost. Thanks to a late night finishing the kitchen, the smell of bleach still burned inside my nose. My fingertips would never be the same after so much scrubbing.

In my right ear, a call continued to ring.

"C'mon, Dad," I murmured, shivering. "I know you're at your desk. You love going to work early in the morning."

A familiar growl made me jump.

"Sheriff. This is Jim."

"Hey! You *are* alive. How are you, Dad?"

"Well, what do you know? It's my favorite daughter."

"Only daughter."

"Same thing."

Grinning, I leaned back in the seat. "Yeah, sorry I've missed our Sunday calls the past couple of weeks."

"Too busy dating that Norman guy to call your father?"

"Nathan."

"Whatever."

I winced. Something about Nathan had pulled me into his orbit like a satellite; everything had revolved around him. I'd missed calls to my family more than once.

"Sorry. I haven't been a very good daughter the past couple of months."

"Don't apologize, kid. I get it. Mark says you're back in the state. When are we going fishing? Then you can stomp around with those big feet, scaring away everything for three miles."

A laugh bubbled out of me. A rush of a dozen childhood memories of fishing with him in the river followed. We spoke about Adventura, repairs in the kitchen, and Mark's current state of easy stress. The sun crept higher, smoothing into long lines of light. Not once did Dad mention Mom.

"Listen, Dad, I talked to Mom yesterday and—"

"Hold on, kid."

The sound of his voice muffled, as if he was covering the mouthpiece. Ten seconds later, he returned.

"Listen, Meg, I gotta go. Can we pick this up later? One of my deputies needs help on a call."

"Sure. Of course. Love you, Dad."

"Love you too."

The line went dead. I dropped my hand to my lap with a sigh. The repercussions of Mom's revelation still flipped my stomach like a roller coaster. I didn't want to think about secrets festering in the shadows of my parents' marriage. But now that Mom had revealed the truth, I couldn't think of anything else.

Memories whirred through my mind. Had there been an undercurrent of tension at Christmas I didn't remember? When had I last spoken with them together? Could I remember the last time I saw them flirting? I came to no solid conclusions.

My thumb hovered over my screen, ready to dial Lexie. I needed *someone* to talk to, but I paused. Deciding against it, I yanked the key free from the engine. The truck groaned when I hopped out and tucked the phone in my pocket.

Just hearing Dad's voice gave me hope. They'd work it—whatever *it* was—out. They had to.

Somehow.

~

THE BACK WHEEL of my shopping cart rattled like the bones of the dead.

I pushed it through the empty aisles of the Pineville Market, ignoring the high-pitched squeak that wailed with every turn. Except for a foggy-eyed cashier, no one else roamed the store.

A sea of fruits and vegetables lured me in. Plump tomatoes. Lumpy carrots with weird knobs. Shiny apples. Crisp pears. My mouth salivated just thinking of tart, tangy huckleberries still warm from the sun. Surely

Adventura had huckleberry bushes. After gathering an assortment of fresh fruits, I slipped to the vegetable section and studied a bag of potatoes.

How many would serve twenty grown males? I grabbed the biggest bag and tossed it in the cart. Cooking for twenty people couldn't be *that* hard. Just a matter of multiplying, really.

I parked by a stand of instant noodles and cracked open Grandma's recipe book that Mom had brought me. Good Morning Muffins—a familiar favorite. Chili and corn bread—too easy. Cupcakes cooked in orange slices —the only recipe I felt confident about. Luckily, Grandma's handwritten bread recipe fell out of the back. I ran a finger down the list of ingredients. Yeast. Flour. Salt. Sugar.

Piece of cake.

In the baking aisle, I squatted down to study the flour bags. Cake flour. All-purpose flour. Bread flour. Pastry flour?

"Geez. What's the difference?"

Opting for the safest route, I chose a bag of all-purpose flour, set it in the cart, and breezed past the brownie mixes. Mom had left behind a double-sized box of brownie mix *just in case,* her note read. *You never know when you'll need brownies in a camp full of men.*

She literally knew everything.

Spices cluttered a shelf in a conglomeration of plastic bottles. The little market couldn't get cell phone reception, but somehow they stocked grapeseed oil. I tossed a few jars of cumin, red pepper flakes, and chili powder in the cart.

Thirty minutes later, I shoved my overflowing cart into the checkout line, passing olive oil, sea salt, celery, a container of hummus, and a wide assortment of other items onto the belt. Mark had tucked $100 cash into the list, so I pulled it out.

The cashier, a thirty-something man with deep-set eyes and a drawn, pale face, scanned my items without speaking. Once he slid the final can of corn across the scanner, he said, "That will be $245.76."

My heart nearly stopped.

"What?"

"Uh ... $245.76."

"It can't be that much."

He licked his lips, gesturing with a limp hand to the bags piled in my cart. "Well..."

"I only have a hundred dollars."

He shrugged and reached for the nearest bag like he had all the time in the world. "Oookay. Then we'll have to return $145.76 worth."

I put a hand out to stop him when he reached for a butternut squash.

"Whoa, buddy. Wait just a second. I need all this food. I'm supposed to feed twenty men."

His expression didn't falter. "And I need $245.76."

"Don't you have coupons? Maybe that'll whittle it down."

"By $145.76?"

"No. But *something*."

He pointed a skinny finger at a sign with a bright yellow star. "Coupons are only for our Star Reward members. Unless they come from the manufacturer. Do you have manufacturer coupons?"

Was he kidding? I'd never used a coupon before, and I hadn't clipped them from the newspaper since third grade.

"No. Where do I find those?"

He shrugged. "Online? The paper?"

"You said reward program?"

"Star Rewards program."

"Great! I'd love to join." I snatched the pen off the check counter. "Where do I sign up?"

An old woman pushed her cart in behind me and started unloading boxes of instant oatmeal. The cashier blew his greasy bangs out of his face and slid a paper filled with squares over the counter. Two minutes later, I slid it back. He picked it up and stared at it through narrowed eyes.

"This address says Jackson City." He peered over the top of the paper.

"It's my parents' address."

"That's not a local address."

I gritted my teeth. "You're right. It's not."

He tossed the paper in the garbage.

"The Star Reward program is only for locals. You'll have to sign up with the Jackson City store to get the deals there. Your total is $245.76."

"Are you kidding?" I cried. "I don't live in Jackson City. I live here."

He pulled another paper from the top of the stack behind the register and set it in front of me.

"Then put your local address this time."

With a growl, I started writing again but stopped. When I looked up at him, he stared past me, deadpan. If I hadn't known any better, I'd have thought he'd fallen asleep with his eyes open. The old lady behind me cleared her throat.

"Um ... I don't know my local address," I said.

His lips bunched. "You don't know your own address?"

"I just moved here two days ago. I'm still trying to figure it all out." He made a move to reach for the paper, but I snatched it back. "No! Don't throw it away again. I'll ... remember in just a second."

"Where is it?"

"Up the canyon."

One of his light blonde eyebrows rose. "You live in the canyon?"

"Yes. *Up* the canyon. At Adventura Boys Camp."

He made a sound in his throat that I couldn't decipher but assumed was disinterest. I made up a road name and put a fake address, then handed it back, daring him to contradict it. He looked from the paper to me, then back to the paper again.

"You remembered?"

"Yep." I slammed the pen down. "4587 Boys Camp Road."

He pointed to the paper. "This says 5478."

"Right. That's what I meant. Just take it. Please?"

He paused, considering, before finally removing the paper and setting the clipboard aside.

"Congratulations," he intoned dully. "You're now a Star Reward program member."

He dashed a plastic card over the scanner and handed it to me. The numbers on the screen whirred for a few seconds. I held my breath, waiting for a forty-or-fifty-dollar discount.

Surely.

"Your new total is $221.17."

"Twenty bucks? That's it?"

He lifted one eyebrow. The old lady let out an exaggerated sigh.

"Fine," I muttered. "Take back the frozen pie crusts and Hot Pockets and Oreos. I'll charge the rest." I pulled out my credit card.

After removing more nonessentials and whittling the total down to $156.29, I rammed my card through the scanner, and the cashier handed me a receipt. Mark would have a fit.

"Have a good day."

I snatched the paper and left. Outside, I slung the groceries into the back of the truck and logged on to my bank account. My heart sank. Subtracting my mortgage and car payment for that month, I only had twenty dollars.

I hadn't been this poor since college.

With a sigh, I climbed into the truck. Maybe working at Adventura Boys Camp wouldn't be the easy vacation I'd hoped for.

~

THE ZOMBIE MOBILE didn't have power steering, so driving had become my new upper-body workout.

Bouncing along the windy canyon road back to Adventura required most of my concentration. The crisp scent of pine filled my nose. Dust billowed in my wake. The river frothed beneath the bridge, swirling in white foam as I barreled across. We'd rafted it once as a family. JJ had fallen in so many times Dad threatened to tie him to the raft. My lips twitched at the memory.

My thoughts spun with abandon while I crept along the dirt road, the cool mountain air whipping through my hair.

Dust the lodge first, I thought. Then sweep. No, unload the groceries. Is the fridge repair guy coming soon? I still haven't mopped. We have no mop. We need more money for basic necessities.

A self-populating list grew in my mind. No matter how much work we sank into the lodge and kitchen, more work popped back up. The first day of camp fast approached. I shifted gears on the truck and wondered what Nathan was doing. Had he moved to New York? Did he miss me yet? I snorted. Probably too busy enjoying his promotion to think about what he'd left behind.

Halfway down the dirt road, the engine chugged, then sputtered. I pressed the gas, but the engine cut out, and the truck lurched to a stop in the middle of the road. Dust ballooned by in puffs.

"Fantastic," I muttered.

I peered at the dashboard. Still had half a tank of gas—or so it said. Who knew if it registered accurately or not. My attempts to resuscitate the engine failed. Not even a click to indicate a turnover. I smacked the steering wheel with my palm, jumping when the horn emitted a wheezy *honk*.

Livid, I elbowed my way out of the old cab and lifted the lid. A conglomeration of rusty pipes, wires, and other ancient architecture peered back at me from under the hood. I grumbled. At least no smoke billowed out. I dropped the hood, blasted by a wave of dust.

My cell phone had limited reception here, but I could walk back to the highway. *Hello, ma'am,* I imagined myself saying to a total stranger after flagging them down. *Can I interest you in driving me an hour out of your way on a dirt road to a summer camp no one's heard about? Thanks.*

My fingers curled into tight fists. There was simply no *time* for this. The staff arrived in the morning. Sweeping and mopping the sprawling lodge floor would take hours alone. Not to mention I had to plan and prep all the meals for the week. Who had time to sit and wait for help?

An idea popped into my head. I swiveled, regarding the long dirt road with new eyes. I could hike back to Adventura.

I hadn't hiked in years. My toes itched to get back on a trail. The sun still hadn't crested the mountains, so the cool air would preserve the groceries for an hour or two. Couldn't be more than an easy four-miler. My fingers tingled at the thought. It had been too long since I'd just ... hiked. Outside. By myself.

"Well," I murmured. "The lodge will have to wait."

After retrieving the truck keys, slinging my backpack over my shoulders, and locking the doors, I left the truck in the middle of the road and headed toward the mountains.

Birds twittered overhead, chasing each other. Sunlight fell in dappled, warm slants through the leaves, shifting with the wind. Every now and then, my foot kicked up a puff of dust. On either side of me, trees rippled up the steep mountain slopes in emerald waves, giving way to chunky boulders and shale fields. The wild excitement of the forest energized my blood. So untamed. So brilliantly fresh.

I stopped in the middle of the road, my head craned back to regard the sky. Something visceral inside me responded to the primitive beauty of the outdoors. I'd forgotten how much I loved it out here. The protection of the peaks. The grandeur of being smaller than everything else. When I slowed down to revel in the sunlight, it all felt right. It had been far too long since I'd lived in the moment. Shucked aside my career expectations in favor of just ... existing.

Maybe I needed to remember the things I loved more often.

Content, I hooked my thumbs in the straps of my backpack and hiked on.

5

FIRST DAY

"B*lister!"*

An explosive *bang* rattled the window above my cot early the next morning. I gasped, rolling off the cot and taking my sleeping bag and pillow with me.

"Mark!" I yelled, grabbing my head when it slammed into the floor. "Why are you screaming?"

"Get up! It's eight o'clock. All the staff members are already here."

I forced my dry eyes open. *What?* The staff was here? Had I overslept? I'd been exhausted from scrubbing the lodge, alphabetizing the spice cupboard, and mouse-proofing the food in the pantry, but I didn't think I'd been *that* exhausted.

"Seriously?"

"We promised them breakfast, Meg. Remember? Eight o'clock?" He tapped on the screen. "Ringabell, sleeping beauty?"

"Crap!" I scrambled to my feet, nearly tripping over the slick sleeping bag. "On my way!"

Within a minute, I donned a pair of jeans, pulled on my official navy-blue Adventura polo, tossed my hair into a messy bun, and headed to the kitchen wearing socks with my Birkenstocks. The sun hid behind the mountains, sending rays of yellow and light pink into the sky. If I hadn't been in such a hurry, I would have stopped to appreciate the early morning grandeur and the sweet scent of dew.

A roar of chattering voices echoed through the lodge and into the kitchen when I rushed inside. The sound of JJ yelling above the collective madness smoothed the noise into a lull, but the chaos resumed with a chorus of laughter.

"Oh man." I threw open the biggest cooler and yanked food out, chucking it onto the counter. "Crap. Crap. Crap. Crap."

My fingers flew, tying a knot in my apron strings as I mentally wrote a to-do list.

"Okay, Megan," I said, closing my eyes. "Think. What do I need to do?"

Slice strawberries. Brown three packages of bacon. Crack, whip, and prep two-dozen eggs for cinnamon French toast. Find cinnamon. Warm syrup without burning it. Did I use butter on the grill? Did I use the whole grill? I could save a fifty-year-old with a blood clot in his lungs, but fixing breakfast for twenty hungry males had me half-paralyzed.

"Curse you, Mark."

We'd argued for thirty minutes the night before about his banned foods list. I'd voted for spinach omelets. They happened to be my forte. He said that we'd insult the gods of eggs with such a dish, and he didn't want to take any chances. With a prayer under my breath, I plunged into preparing his favorite: French toast.

Ten minutes later, I cracked my tenth egg while simultaneously attempting—with little success—to turn on the grill. A strange clicking sound came from it every now and then, but nothing happened. When I reached for another egg, my fingertips slid into something gooey. Glancing down, I recoiled. Nestled among the whole eggs in the carton lay four gleaming egg yolks. I must have accidentally cracked them open over the carton while I fiddled with the grill.

"You have got to be kidding me."

I plucked the yolks out of the carton, lobbing them into the bowl. They slid down the side, breaking in a lemony mudslide.

Except for a shuffling noise coming from beneath the grill, further attempts to light it met with failure. In desperation, I flipped the ovens on, praying that French toast could be baked. Preferably in less than ten minutes.

Mark called my name as I hacked strawberries into uneven chunks. He popped into the room through the swinging door, forehead creased. Strawberry juice stained my fingers.

"Yeah?"

"Something is smelling a bit funky. Is that on fire?"

I whirled around to find smoke curling off the grill. The scent of char lingered in the air.

"Ha! You do work, you rotten monster!"

"So, nothing is on fire?"

"Not yet."

He disappeared a little too eagerly. I grabbed the package of bacon and unloaded the whole thing. Bacon would be a great place to start. The high-pitched chattering began again, but with more intensity. I opened the oven to make sure it had started to warm. A brown streak leaped out of the darkness, heading right for my face. I screamed and fell to the ground. The fluffy tail and beady eyes of a squirrel stared back at me before the creature darted underneath the island.

No. Way.

"Hey!" I screamed, throwing a metal spoon at it. "Get out of here!"

I scrambled to my feet, grabbing a broom propped against the wall. Two metal bowls clattered off the shelf. Startled by the resounding *bang* of metal on the tile floor, the squirrel bolted to the fridge and shimmied behind it.

"Out!" I screeched. "Out of my kitchen!"

I shoved the broomstick behind the fridge, swinging it wildly. A picture fell off the wall and hit the floor with a crack, sending glass shards across the tile. Seconds later, the frantic clicking abated. When I looked up, the squirrel stood on top of the fridge, frozen, all four legs splayed out.

"Get outta here!"

With the end of the broom, I shoved the screen door open. The squirrel leaped onto the ground, rushed out the door, and hurtled up a nearby tree.

"Meg?"

"Is everything all right?"

"Has a meteor hit?"

Mark and JJ stood in the doorway. Mark's mouth hung open. JJ rolled his lips together.

"There was a damn squirrel in the oven!"

"No way!" Mark said, laughing. "I thought I heard something."

JJ sniffed. "Is something burning?"

"The bacon!"

With a mad dash—and the crunch of glass beneath my feet—I hurried over to the grill and attacked the fried pork with a metal spatula. Remnants of black meat stuck to the grill. Some pieces were charred, others barely warm. Obviously, the grill wasn't the most consistent surface.

"Blister," Mark said, "do you need any—"

"Fine!" I called over my shoulder. "I'm fine. I'll get it out in just a second. Just need a ... a few more minutes!"

First day, I told myself. All first days at all jobs are tough. I can cook breakfast. This isn't that hard.

Once I freed the charred bacon and flipped it around the half-heated grill, I cleared space on one side and tossed on slices of French toast in rows. My post-squirrel hysteria calmed enough for me to think straight.

"I got this," I said to myself, taking deep, cleansing yoga breaths. "I got this."

While the French toast bubbled on the grill, I reached for a plate. My hand landed on an empty shelf. I fumbled around. Nothing. A horrifying thought occurred to me. I tore through the pantry and the other cupboards.

"I forgot plates!" I said, running a hand through my hair. "Oh, no!"

How could I have forgotten to buy plates? *Oh, well. No way to fix it now.* They'd have to eat with their hands.

Ten minutes later, I stared at a pile of half-cooked, half-charred French toast. Random hot spots on the grill led to the toast being burned or soggy. No in between existed.

Hoping the staff would either like burnt food or wouldn't notice the squishy middles, I placed the French toast in a mixing bowl below a rolling window that opened into the dining area. It groaned when I tugged on the rope that pulled it up. Twenty pairs of eyes turned to stare at me.

"And that," Mark said from where he stood on top of a table, "is Megan, your lovely chef. She doubles as a squirrel hunter, everyone. Let her know if you need help. Give her a round of applause."

A chorus of mumbled greetings and half-hearted claps came at me. I waved, wondering, based on their strange expressions, what I must have looked like. When I reached down to smooth the apron, my fingers ran over an eggshell.

"Meg," Mark said with a fixed smile, tapping his thumb against his leg. "Is, uh, breakfast ready?"

"Oh, yeah. Uh ... the first round of French toast is done." I forced a smile. "Help yourself."

The crowd surged forward as one. Just as the first staff member approached, my heart stopped a second time. I froze. I'd forgotten to fix the plate dilemma. And where was the syrup? Of course there was syrup. There had to be syrup. What kind of a fool would forget *syrup*? My mind spun back to the grocery store. Surely, I hadn't forgotten...

Yes. I had.

"Where are the plates?"

"Is there any syrup?"

My tongue turned into a packet of sand. The whole crowd stared while I mentally fumbled for a way out. Was French toast palatable without syrup? Probably not *this* French toast.

"Ah ... no," I said. "No syrup. Forgive me, I should have explained. This isn't just regular French toast. This is, ah, special."

A burly Tongan—Sione, if I remembered correctly from the twins' adventures in California—lifted up a piece, studying it with sharp brown eyes.

"Sure smells like regular French toast." He tore into it with a savage bite. "Tastes like it." He grimaced. "Kinda."

The thick, smoky scent of bacon wafted past me. At least I'd managed to get that right.

"Haven't you heard of French toast and bacon sandwiches?" I asked. "No? Oh, well, allow me to enlighten you. It's ... the latest rave in breakfast food. Instead of a sweet, er, breakfast theme, salty's in."

I plucked a piece of French toast from the pile and waved it around, ignoring their suspicious stares. A few dots of liquid egg splashed the counter.

"Load it up with bacon, add a bit of butter, and voila!" I shoved two pieces of bacon between slices with a beaming smile. The gooey middles smushed beneath my fingers, and egg ran down the back of my hand. "A delicious breakfast sandwich with lots of protein."

"What are the strawberries for?" someone asked.

"That's the sweet variation. You just put powdered sugar and strawberries in the sandwich instead of bacon. There you have it. Breakfast sandwiches without the stickiness of syrup."

"What do we put them on?"

"There's no plates."

"Oh," I said, waving an airy hand toward a roll of paper towels. "No need for plates with just sandwiches. We're ... going green. Conserving water. Just use a paper towel."

Mark glared at me from the back, nostrils flaring. *Are you kidding?* he mouthed. I ignored him.

With a few hesitant shrugs, the staff stepped forward, ramming bacon and strawberries between their pieces of French toast. I waited, breath held, for someone to call me out as a fraud. But they moved through the line with nods of thanks. Only a couple of them seemed overly suspicious.

Grateful for a chance to step away, I returned to the grill and started slinging more French toast on the heated surface. The whir of the overhead fan drowned out the chatter of the staff in the background. I closed my eyes.

One meal down, I thought. One hundred seventy-nine more to go.

6

YOU ARE GIRL POWER

My salvation arrived by phone call.

After the disaster of my first breakfast, I paced around the kitchen, wiping down the already gleaming stainless-steel countertops. *No syrup? No plates? A squirrel?* The depth of my disbelief could not be measured.

The vibration of my phone almost didn't break through my haze of embarrassment. I pulled my phone out of my back pocket and saw Lexie's name. I hesitated but finally pressed it to my ear.

"Hey, Lex."

"Hey!" she said. "You answered! How long have you been gone? Like two weeks?"

"Two days."

She groaned. "I'm. Going. To. Die."

I paused, my mouth half-open, debating whether I should share my horrible morning. Or, more correctly, the struggle of the past two days. She'd be marrying Bradley soon, and that gave me an unexpected hesitation.

"You still there?" she asked.

"Oh, yes. Sorry." I leaned back against a counter.

"So," she drawled. "How is it?"

I swallowed, my eyes scanning the kitchen in two short seconds. *What am I doing here?* I should have been in a new hospital, placing an IV or paging a cardiologist. I'd jumped in over my head.

"It's, ah ... it's..."

"That bad?"

My shoulders slumped. I couldn't hold it in. "Yes! It's been crazy. Lex, you won't even believe what just happened. My Mom fell apart, and there isn't any money for food, and I forgot *syrup*. Who forgets syrup? Oh! And there are squirrels in my oven. Squirrels."

"Sounds like a bad pregnancy joke."

"Lexie!"

"Sorry. Couldn't help myself. Tell me what's going on. Squirrels in paradise? Okay, now it just sounds like a bad rap song."

Recounting the breakfast fiasco took ten minutes. "A squirrel?" she asked, giggling. "Oh, Megan. I'm *dying*."

"It was horrible." I dragged a hand through my hair. "But, okay. It's kind of funny, too."

"Horrible would have been if the squirrel bit you."

"True," I said, laughing. "Very true."

"How are the staff?"

I thought of their perplexed expressions. "Who knows? It's hard to tell. I mean, I served them French toast without plates or syrup right after chasing a squirrel. I think my first impression went over like a snowball in hell."

Lexie giggled. "Another great rap song."

I chuckled with her until the reality of my situation nudged its way back in like a shadow. "Lex," I said, sobering. "I don't belong here. I miss work. I miss being a nurse."

I miss you, I wanted to say.

My heart longed for the hospital. The sound of my badge swishing against my scrubs. Doctors calling for me with new orders. Connecting with a patient. Calming someone who felt as if their world had turned upside down. It all felt so much more intense and important than flipping bacon.

"Too bad. You can't come home. Look at it this way—it will be good for you to do something you aren't uber-talented at. I, for one, am devastated I didn't see the Great Squirrel Chase. Oh, I'm going to pee. I have to stop thinking about it."

While she alternated between snorting and recounting snippets of my morning, I picked at a loose thread on my shirt. Leaving everything behind had turned out to be harder than I'd expected. I even missed my down comforter and my sugar cookie candle. I may as well have moved to another planet.

With indifferent natives.

"C'mon," Lexie said. "Don't wallow, Meg. It's not like you. It's only been two days."

Outside, Justin strode by carrying an armful of firewood on his shoulder, squinting as he stared into the sun. "Yeah, well, you wouldn't believe how beautiful the scenery is up here," I said, tracking him as he disappeared around the side of the lodge.

"Have you heard from Nathan?"

"No."

"Think you will?"

"Hope not. Any news with you and Bradley?"

"He hasn't proposed in the years since you left, if that's what you mean. Nothing new to report, really. I just wanted to hear your voice. We already miss you."

"I miss you, too."

Lexie's voice softened. "You got this, Meg. It probably won't be easy, but you're Megan. You *are* girl power. You can do anything. You know? There may be a few growing pains, but you'll figure it out."

Sighing, I gazed out the window. Branches swayed in the wind. I didn't know how to cook for twenty people. I wasn't familiar with most of the recipes, and I had a suspicious feeling I'd be at war with a squirrel, a grill, and an oven. To make matters worse, the fridge still didn't work, and I wasn't sure when to start piecing together lunch. Or if it would be eaten. My easy summer in the trees was slipping out of my grasp already, and camp hadn't even started.

But Lexie was right.

"Yeah," I said, blowing out a hot breath. "You're right."

"Duh. I'm also late for work and have to go. Good luck, Meg. Sounds like you're going to need it."

Mark's Banned Food List.
(Blister: This. Is. Serious.)

- *Egg White Omelettes*
- *Gluten substitutes. We love gluten. Keep the gluten!*
- *Kale. Don't EVEN*
- *Light Ranch. Light anything*
- *Skim milk*
- *Fat-free anything*
- *Turkey sausage*
- *Brown rice.*
- *Quinoa. Don't try to fool me again.*

Saturday and Sunday slid by in a blur of dusty shoes, cheap new plates, and the stress of cooking for twenty grown men. Thanks to a temperamental oven, meals didn't go well. My first attempts at homemade bread remained straight dough in the middle, while the edges firmed up to the consistency of a clay pot. The bland chili received no applause.

Luckily, the buzz of preparation spread across all of Adventura, keeping everyone too busy to care about boring food. By late Sunday night, camp glimmered like a crystal. Except the kitchen, which still needed a bulldozer. I fell asleep the moment I closed my eyes and woke what seemed like ten minutes later.

"Rise and shine, Adventura," Mark sang Monday morning in a dramatic operetta over a loudspeaker. "The campers will arrive soon."

Thirty minutes later, the scent of simmering gravy and fresh biscuits filled the lodge with warmth. The staff mingled in the background. Snippets of conversation floated into the kitchen as I tossed plates, napkins, and silverware onto the counter.

"Finally," I murmured to myself, sliding two trays of fresh, doughy biscuits into separate ovens. "A hot, yummy breakfast on the first day of camp. On plates, no less." The oven doors banged shut. "Nailed it."

Five minutes later, Justin stepped through the swinging door wearing a dusty pair of work pants and heavy boots.

"Hey, Meg. Need some help?"

I glanced up from where I crouched at the fridge, rummaging for a box of butter. His denim blue eyes cut right through mine.

"Uh ... sure. Will you check the biscuits for me? They should only be halfway done by now, but that oven is almost as grumpy as the squirrel I evicted."

Forcing myself to look away from his rugged attractiveness didn't come easy, but I returned to my search for butter. Did he tousle his hair on purpose, or was it wild from the intermittent wind? I couldn't imagine him caring about his hair.

"Uh, Meg?"

I popped back out from the bowels of the fridge. The uncertainty in his voice made my stomach drop.

"Yeah?"

"I think they're done."

A tray of round, blackened discs emerged from the oven. My mouth dropped. "Seriously? I just barely put them in!"

In two steps, I reached the second oven door and yanked it open. A tentative, weak wave of heat billowed out. Even though the second oven was set at the same temperature, these biscuits still had a doughy shine.

"Fabulous." I slammed the door shut again. "We'll just give the staff bowls of gravy to eat."

He eyed the gravy pan. Generous lumps clumped around the edges, but he wisely said nothing.

"Look on the bright side," Justin said as he slid the burned tray of biscuits on top of the grill. "No rabid squirrel. You have plates. And these will make excellent baseballs. You are three steps ahead of your first day."

"If you have a bat, I know exactly what I want to do with it," I muttered, glaring at the stove.

He laughed and headed for the door.

"Just set out cold cereal for them to fill up on if the other biscuits don't turn out. It's a fitting tribute to the first day of camp, don't you think?"

No, I wanted to growl, but after seeing his illuminating smile, I couldn't bring myself to be too angry. The gravy had a weird texture anyway.

With a sigh, I headed for the pantry.

AFTER BREAKFAST, Adventura lay quiet and peaceful.

The lodge door creaked in the soft breeze. Staff members buzzed around camp, charged with energy.

The tranquility shattered with the sound of a car horn. Within minutes, the woods teemed with adolescent boys threatening to string underwear up the flagpole. Twenty minutes after check-in, two boys were unaccounted for, three couldn't find their bags, and five parents had forgotten to sign waivers. Mark moved amongst the pandemonium with ease, barking orders like a commander as his voice faded in and out of the radio static.

Two counselors and at least four campers inhabited each campsite. This year, Mark had employed ten counselors to manage five campsites. The rest of the staff directed camp programs, like white-water rafting and crafts. JJ was in charge of the climbing wall. Sione and a blond surfer named Hollis oversaw the waterfront. And an aging, soft-spoken ex-army infantry officer, Gary, led the rifle and archery ranges. Wires of curly, black hair streaked with white sprouted from his head, and a pearly smile that contrasted with his dark skin filled his face whenever he saw me.

JJ and I stood in the lodge, watching the pandemonium with detached amusement. At least we didn't have to be out there.

"Did breakfast seem weird to you?" I asked, leaning back against a table.

"Yep."

"So, it wasn't just me? It was tense, right?"

"Yep."

"Why?"

"Because there wasn't enough food."

My heart sank. "Really? I thought they had enough."

"There was enough cold cereal for one bowl each, yes. And the biscuits broke one of my teeth, and the gravy was lumpier than a mattress. So, let's just say the food was ... underwhelming."

"Told you to go for cold cereal like the rest of them."

His upper lip curled up over his teeth.

"Right," I muttered. "More cold cereal next week."

Mark had bought plastic plates, trays, cups, and utensils from the dollar store with his personal credit card over the weekend. Based on his harried expression when he returned, he had debt problems far bigger than mine.

JJ grimaced over his coffee mug. "Although you pulled a smooth one with the whole no-syrup-French-toast thing, they aren't as stupid as they look. They know you just forgot."

I scowled. "Wonderful."

"It's not a bad thing, Megara. Just own it."

The low thud of boots on the back porch preceded a knock on the screen door, jarring me from my spiral of embarrassment.

"Come in," I called. "You don't have to knock."

Troy, a fiery redhead with the corded arms of a swimmer, stepped into the kitchen. His pale green eyes reminded me of sea foam. Freckles dotted every visible part of his skin, even the back of his neck.

JJ jerked his head in greeting. "Hey, Troy."

"Hey," Troy said, wiping his palm on his pant leg. He turned to me. "Uh, I came to introduce myself."

I stuck out my hand with a warm smile. "I'm Megan."

He accepted my hand, shaking with a firm grip. "Mark hired me as the medical officer. Just graduated with my EMT certification. He mentioned that you're a nurse, right?"

"Yes. I worked—uh, I came from a Cardiac Intensive Care Unit."

At my accidental stumble, JJ's gaze flickered to me and back to his magazine.

Troy studied his shoes like they were about to swallow him. "So, uh ... can I ask you questions if something comes up? I don't have a lot of experience."

"Sure. Swing by whenever. The door's always open."

His bunched shoulders smoothed out a little. "Oh," he said. "Great. Thanks."

"Anytime."

Troy let out a long, relieved breath once he stepped onto the porch, and he whistled as he strode away. I watched him go.

"See?" I pointed to the door. "That was awkward, right? But he wasn't that awkward when he was talking with the other guys this morning. I know. I watched."

"That's creepy."

"It's not creepy. It's ... awareness."

JJ turned a page and yawned. "Yeah," he said. "You're right. He was a mess just now."

"Don't they like me?"

"Oh," he drawled with a sly smile, "I don't think that's the problem. Welcome to Manland. Strange culture, I grant you. But you'll figure it out. Get them really full." His face twisted in thought. "And more meat. Whatever you do, make more meat."

I eyed him. "Aren't you vegetarian?"

"*I* am. Everyone else isn't. I'll make my own breakfast so you don't have to worry about it. I don't mind."

"Thanks, JJ."

Once he departed for the climbing tower, Grandma's recipe book seemed to stare at me from the kitchen. I straightened up. I *did* make a wicked pan of brownies. Perhaps their friendship just needed a little ... chocolate.

Mark rushed into the kitchen, breathless and red-faced, just as I reached for the recipe book.

"Hey, blister, uh ... I totally forgot something really, really important."

"Oh?"

"You don't happen to have a food handler's permit, do you?"

I snapped my fingers. "Left it at home with my hairnet and apron."

His glare cut a hot line through me. "I need you to go into town and get it. Right now. Like ... don't fix any more food until you have it. I forgot to have you do it before you came. It's my fault."

"Where do I go?" I asked.

He pulled a folded piece of paper out of the back of his Clipboard of Power. "Here's the information. Find a place with wi-fi in Pineville, and take it there. Print off two copies. And maybe backdate it to before camp started?"

With a snort, I accepted the paper. "What about lunch?"

"Set out stuff for sandwiches. We can throw it all together."

I beamed. Best day ever!

"Sounds great!"

He paused halfway out the door. "Oh, and Meg? Don't fail the test. Just ... get all the answers right."

He disappeared before I could counter with a witty quip. I shoved the recipe book to the back of the counter. Brownies—and the rampant adoration of the staff—would have to wait until dinner.

DINNER SNUCK up on me like a bandit.

By the time I showered, set out food for lunch, tracked down the truck keys, and drove down the canyon, eleven o'clock had come and gone. I hunkered down at an Italian restaurant that smelled like garlic. A middle-aged woman with tomato sauce on her shirt let me print the certificates.

"We're all family here," she said, waving off my profuse gratitude.

Four o'clock rolled around as I climbed out of the truck back at camp, food handler's permit in hand. Spaghetti, French bread, salad, and meat sauce had to be ready at five. I jogged through camp, spilling into the empty kitchen with my heart racing.

Brownies and epicness forthcoming. Win their hearts tonight, Meg, I reminded myself. Win. Their. Hearts.

After slinging meat into the pans, filling a massive pot with water, and firing up the stove, I tossed two extra packages of noodles in the boiling pot and cooked twice as much ground beef as I'd originally planned. These twenty hungry men would leave the lodge stuffed like Thanksgiving turkeys.

By the time I leaned outside and rang the dinner bell, the buttered pasta waited in a gleaming, piping-hot bowl. Meat sauce bubbled on the stovetop in three separate pans, and I'd knelt on the floor in front of the oven to watch the French bread brown to perfection. The smell of brownies drifted through the air like a tease. Several curious noses sniffed through the swinging door.

By the time the staff lined up to eat, sweat ringed my underarms, my face flushed as hot as the stovetop, and I wanted to shove my head into a cooler of ice. I satisfied myself with standing at the now-working freezer with the door open.

"Dinner looks great, Meg," Justin said, gliding by with a fist extended.

"Solid work."

"Thanks." I bumped our fists. "Feeling good about this one."

"Busy day?"

I put a hand to my high ponytail. "No. I always look like this."

He chortled, shoving through the swinging door and into the lodge. Over his shoulder, my eyes caught empty tables and chairs. I straightened. *Hold up.* Where was everyone? I hurried to the window and counted heads. Ten. Why were there only ten guys?

"Hey." I hurried after Justin, grabbing his arm. The tips of my fingers sank slightly into his skin. I let go, taking a step back. "Oh, sorry. Uh ... where is everyone? Are they coming late? I can keep it warm." I frowned. "I think."

Justin's brows furrowed. He lifted an arm, gesturing to the room.

"This is everyone."

"Whoa!" Mark cried, coming out of the kitchen behind Sione and Hollis. "Are we feeding the Salvation Army tonight, blister? Why so much food?"

I sucked in a sharp breath, reassessing every face. Program staff. The only people gathered tonight were program staff. I swallowed.

"The counselors eat with the campers, right?" I asked.

Justin bit his bottom lip as if he sensed where this disaster was about to go. "Yes. The counselors teach the campers to cook over a fire. That's why the commissary distributes food to them."

"Right." I gave a cool thumbs-up. "*Right.* That's what I thought. Just checking."

He eyed me askance but said nothing as he reached for a plate. I'd just made enough spaghetti for the whole staff—twenty people—when I only had to cook for ten. I smiled at everyone as they passed through the kitchen into the lodge.

Leftovers for days!

Mark sped through announcements for the program staff while they ate, discussing the schedule for the next day while I cut through the brownies, stacking them in a perfect formation on the plate. Only half the spaghetti had disappeared, leaving mounds behind. JJ sent me a thumbs-up.

As nonchalantly as possible, I set brownies out at each table and retreated back to the kitchen to wait.

Rampant adoration, here we come, I thought.

One by one, the program staff polished off the brownies. Just as the last brownie disappeared, all of them stood at Mark's call.

"Let's go, ladies," Mark said. "We have a night hike to run."

"Thanks for the brownies, Megan," Sione called. A few other staff waved. They shuffled out the front of the lodge, guffawing and chortling with each other. *What?* I wanted to say. *That's it?*

I sighed. *So much for rampant adoration.* I grabbed a corner piece out of the pan. At least the brownies had been edible.

The kitchen door slammed open, and Mark ran inside, brownie in hand. He clapped me on the shoulder.

"Dinner was awesome tonight, blister. Seriously. We needed a good carb load before the night hike. It can't be easy trying to figure out how to cook for that many people or getting stuck in this hot room with a lot of dishes to do. So, thank you."

Suspicious, I narrowed my eyes just enough to study him.

"What?"

"Dinner," he said, enunciating. "It was great. Thank you."

My tense arms unwound.

"Really?"

"Yeah." He chucked me lightly on the shoulder. "I'm really glad you came. Thanks for all you're doing."

"But I—"

He shook his head, cutting me off. "Nope. No buts. I'm just glad you came." His radio crackled. "Do you want to come on the night hike?"

"I need to clean up."

"You can do that later."

The idea of a warm bed and a good, long sleep pulled at me. My legs still ached from a brief morning run with JJ.

"Next time," I said. "Otherwise, I'll be scrubbing tomato sauce for hours tomorrow."

With a shrug, he spun on his heels and headed out the back door, letting the screen slam shut behind him. I stood there, feeling a strange bundle in my chest, both light and heavy, confusing and clear, at the same time.

7

THE RIGHT TIME

Wednesday morning, lodgepole pines flashed by the truck like thousands of matchsticks topped with green branches. I'd set out bowls, spoons, oatmeal, and milk for breakfast before escaping, leaving only a quick note of explanation for Mark.

Running to Pineville for groceries.

The wind whipped my hair around my face as I navigated the winding canyon, interspersed with sharp boulders and a frothy river. My thoughts grew as wide as the canyon until I reined them back in at the Frolicking Moose Cafe.

A wave of coffee and vanilla bean greeted me when I stepped inside. Real hardwood floors gleamed in the honey-glow of several lamps. "Welcome to the Frolicking Moose," a barista with burnished copper hair and porcelain skin said. "My name is Lizbeth. Wi-fi password is on the chalkboard. Can I get you something to drink?"

She pitched a white washcloth over her shoulder. It landed right on the spigot.

"Basketball player?" I asked.

"Nah. I just practice when no one's here. Do you work at Adventura?"

My eyebrows shot up.

"Yeah, I do. How'd you know?"

She flashed me a quick grin, her eyes sparkling. "I'm in touch with the forest spirits, but I'm not crazy. I reserve that designation for people like my mother." Her playful gaze and layers of hair reminded me of a fairy. Young. Bright. Willowy. And a tad bit quirky.

"You've heard of Adventura?"

"JJ and Mark bum off the internet all the time. You have to be their sister. Your eyes are just like JJ's."

"That's a compliment, right?"

Her lips twitched. "Trust me," she said, turning away. "Looking like JJ is a blessing from the gods. Let me know if you want anything."

She wandered back to the counter, the layers of her summery white dress trailing behind her. Four text messages from Lexie occupied my attention while I waited for the wi-fi to connect.

Found out they make birthday cake Oreos now. Saboteurs.

The gym is boring without you showing up the male lifters.

Bought a Prana headband. Look like a dork. I long for sculpted cheekbones.

Still not engaged. The suspense is killing me.

After responding to Lexie and a text message from Dad to schedule a Rudy's Diner date, I switched to my internet browser. "Let's check on Nathan," I murmured and logged onto Facebook.

Lexie had posted a meme about donuts, a friend from college had sent me a message, and Nathan...

...had posted a lovely photo of his new flat in New York.

An ache in my chest made me grimace, but it ebbed away. His profile betrayed nothing about our broken relationship. Had I wanted it to? Not really. But some acknowledgment of my slip from his life would have been nice. At least, I thought it would.

Resigned, I switched to email. A bill payment reminder from Travelers Credit Card caught my eye. Right below it waited for a message from an unfamiliar sender.

"Jodie Renner?" I murmured, clicking on it.

Megan,

My name is Jodie Renner. I work with EveryHealth Corporation as a nurse recruiter. Your old manager, Karen, speaks highly of you.

If you're still looking for a job, give me a call or send me an email. I have lots of options. No reason to limit yourself to the Intensive Care Units. We even take travel-nursing contracts. I can direct you to the right companies if you'd like.

EveryHealth has been on a building binge the last decade, so I have contacts everywhere. I think I could find you a flight-nurse slot. Karen mentioned you've been on that path. Would that interest you?

I look forward to hearing from you.

Regards,

Jodie

A scour pad moved underneath my ribs with every breath. As soon as I finished reading the email, I set my phone down, blinking.

I think I could find you a flight-nurse slot.

Would that interest you?

The thought made my heart pound in my throat. A flight-nurse position would mean classes. Certifications. New thrills. A chance to exceed expectations. Major career advancement. It seemed too good to be true. Too easy.

"You still on planet earth?"

Lizbeth's voice broke me out of my trance. I jumped.

"Whoa, Nessie." She held up a palm. "Take it easy. Just wanted to make sure you weren't having one of those weird seizures where people just stare."

"No," I said with a sheepish smile. "I'm good. Just ... thinking."

She put her palms on the counter and leaned against them. "Want to talk about it? Baristas make better therapists than bartenders. I kept the Olsens from divorcing last year."

"It's more of a career thing than a relationship thing."

Lizbeth's eyebrows rose.

"Oh?"

"Uh ... just a job opportunity may be coming through. Seems a little too good to be true, though."

Her pixie-like expression fell. "Probably is." The bell on the door tinkled. A man with a belt buckle the size of my face swaggered in, cowboy boots thudding with every step. Lizbeth backed away from me.

"Good luck." She waved a pale hand. "I hope it's something good."

"Yeah. Me too."

But something good at the right time, I silently thought. What if Jodie found me a job while I was working at Adventura? Could I leave if the perfect position came up?

Deciding I'd think about that later—if Jodie could even work such magic—I flipped my phone over, pulled up the email, and tapped out a quick response. I doubted she could simply wave a wand and find me a flight-nurse job.

But maybe.

Jodie,

I'm very interested. When can you talk?

—Megan Bailey

Things That Scare Me

- ~~*Choking when I'm alone.*~~
- ~~*Rustling in the forest.*~~
- ~~*Mark with a gleam in his eye.*~~
- ~~*Current politics.*~~
- *Not being a flight-nurse.*
- *Mom when she cries.*
- ~~*Drowning*~~

THE FIRST WEEK ended like a slow bleed. By the end, everyone—even the campers—looked haggard, sunburned, and exhausted. When the last camper left at nine on Saturday morning, the staff scattered to Pineville and Jackson City. JJ and I stayed behind. I dropped onto his cot in the cabin he shared with Mark and stared at a picture of El Capitan he'd tacked on the wall.

"Hey," he said, looking up from adjusting a climbing harness. "Just you and me, huh?"

"Yep."

"Just the way I like it," he murmured.

I grabbed a plush basketball from the floor and attempted to throw it in the hoop. It missed and bounced off the wall. A vibration buzzed against my leg, and I pulled out my phone to see a voicemail reminder from earlier this morning. While JJ studied the tension on his harness, I clicked on the voicemail and pressed the phone to my ear. It crackled at first but came through clearly when I sat up.

"Megan Bailey, this is Jameson from Traveler's Credit Card. I'm calling in regards to a missed payment for last month—"

My heart skipped. I shut the phone off and stuffed it under my leg. The credit card bill. I'd completely forgotten. My mortgage and car payment would have already gone through by now, leaving only twenty dollars in my account.

Dad, I thought with a sudden spark of hope. *I'll ask him for a small loan at lunch next week. Problem solved.*

"Hey, wanna prank Mark?" I asked, shoving thoughts of debt aside. "We could string his underwear up the flagpole."

JJ snorted. "Rookie."

"Maybe a run? I want to build my endurance back up."

He tossed a harness over to me. It landed on my chest with a heavy *thud*. "We'll go for a run this evening. Get your shoes. We're climbing."

I perked up. "Where?"

"It's a surprise."

After we burdened ourselves with ropes, carabiners, and gear, JJ strode into the forest, his man bun bobbing with every step. He wore a pair of gray shorts and a loose white shirt that deepened his already tan skin. The bulging muscles of his calves flexed with every step.

"Where are we going?" I asked, glancing behind us. "The tower is that way."

"We're not climbing the tower."

Content to be away from Adventura and alone with JJ, I followed with no further questions. JJ had a soothing, easy presence—the perfect counter to Mark's constant spark of energy. Sunlight rippled through the leaves as we passed underneath the branches. The path gave way to a trail, then a footpath. I'd just started to work up a sweat when we stopped.

"This," JJ said, craning his head back, "is what we're going to climb."

A wall of rock stood before us, decorated by occasional spurts of grass. Tufts of wildflowers clung to ledges barely wide enough for a handhold. The top loomed far overhead. The sun blazed full on my shoulders now, and I enjoyed the friendly burn.

I dropped the rope I'd been carrying. The climb would be two rope lengths, I imagined. A nice challenge to get back into it. JJ would lead. He always did. I stretched my arms behind my neck.

"Perfect. Let's scale this beast."

JJ morphed into another man when he climbed. Gone were the carefree smiles, the easygoing nature, and the universal acceptance. His face grew taut. His eyes hardened. He glanced back at me over his shoulder, clips swinging at his hips.

"Ready?"

"On belay, brother."

We committed to silence for the next half hour, except for the occasional comment as JJ searched for handholds. He ascended with a fluid, easy grace, taking his time. He made it look so natural, as if he'd been born on the rocks.

Once at the top of the first pitch, he called down.

"Let's go, Megara. Your turn."

I ran my fingers along the harness to keep it from digging into my thighs. "Right," I said, cracking my neck. "Here I come."

Within two minutes, my feet stumbled over the footholds. Although I burrowed deep with my toe box, my shoes didn't grip like JJ's. Undaunted, I pressed on, moving from grip to grip, using the power in my legs. If nothing else, pushing my body released some of my simmering frustration. For the second time since arriving at Adventura, I lived in the moment and let go of the rest.

When I grappled for the top, my arms weak with fatigue and legs trembling, JJ grabbed my arm. He pulled me up, and I flopped onto my back.

"You're weak sauce, Megara." He tossed me a Nalgene with a grin. "Looks like we'll have to climb together every weekend until you get your strength back."

"Shut. Up," I muttered in between pants. The muscles in both my hands had started to cramp. I shook them out. One of my nails pulsed. I'd chipped it so deep it bled. JJ sat back and stared at the view. I straightened up, leaning back on my palms, and gazed over the mountains.

"Oh. Wow."

"Yeah." He pulled a long draw of water. "I know."

Fields of evergreen trees rippled below us, interspersed with bulwarks of stone. The sun hadn't risen above the mountains yet, shedding folds of light on the ravines and cliffs across from us. Wispy strung-cotton clouds filled the wedge of cerulean sky. We loomed above Adventura, gazing down like nesting eagles. The folds of the mountain cradled us in their deep grooves. Standing on top of something made me feel powerful and alive in a way that made my blood buzz. Cocooned in my job and Midwest world, I'd forgotten how good it felt to be part of a mountain.

"It's incredible, isn't it?" I breathed. "Some people are still asleep at home. And here we are ... standing on top of the world."

"We're the lucky ones," he said. "We live here."

We sat close together, soaking in the majesty of the mountains until JJ broke the silence. He leaned back, scuffing his shoes on loose slate.

"So, you spent some time with Mom last week. What do you think?"

"What do you mean?"

He stared into the distance, his jaw tight. "Something's off. I've only been back from California for a month, but Mom and Dad are ... different. The whole vibe is weird. Mark shrugged it off when I asked him. Said it wasn't his business."

I swallowed, recalling with frightening clarity the fear in Mom's eyes. The way she trembled when I hugged her. Her desperate need for privacy and connection all at the same time.

"Define 'weird.'" I chucked a rock off the ledge. "Mom and Dad used to dance to Neil Diamond in the kitchen, remember? When it comes to parents, 'weird' is subjective."

He shook his head. "I don't think they're talking. Dad hardly ever comes around. Mom texts me all the time about the stupidest stuff. She tried to hide it, but when she found out you were going to come, she cried. I don't know, Meg. Something is up."

My throat ached with the desire to tell him. *Why should he be the only one who doesn't know?* But my promise to Mom held me back.

"What if something *were* up?" I asked. "That doesn't mean it's the end of the world. Right? I mean ... what do you think it would even mean?"

His nostrils flared. "I don't know. The end of the family?"

I recoiled. "What?"

"If Mom and Dad were having marriage issues, everything would fall apart."

"How?"

"They're supposed to be the glue. Mom is always successful. Flight-nurse. Marathoner. Tri-athlete. She doesn't fail at anything. What does it mean that she is—if my assumption is correct—failing the most important relationship of her life?"

His words hit too close to something hot and painful inside me. It prickled up my throat like a moving porcupine. A thousand thoughts whirled through my mind at top speed. Was it failure? All I managed to say was, "No one is indomitable, JJ. She'd be furious if she knew you thought she was. That sets an expectation that's almost impossible to maintain."

JJ swallowed, and I wondered what he wasn't saying.

"Are you more afraid of what it would mean for them, or for you?" I asked.

He paused. "I don't know."

"I've been texting Dad. We're planning on meeting up for lunch soon."

He shrugged, twisting his lips. For a moment, a flash of pain illuminated his eyes, then disappeared. I wondered if Dad had made room for JJ the way he'd made room for me.

Another long silence passed. JJ fell into a brooding stare while I attempted to navigate the awkward waters of what I knew and he didn't. No matter how I imagined a conversation that might comfort him, they all ended with me breaking my promise to Mom.

I nudged JJ with my elbow. "I'm sure things will be fine," I said. "Maybe they just need some space. They've been together forever, you know? They belong together."

"Yeah." He twirled a leaf in his hand, then flicked it to the side. "Maybe."

"You always have Mark and me."

His eyes met mine. They'd hardened into olive-green steel but softened at the edges. "Yeah?" he asked with a wry grin.

"Yeah. Always."

The intensity of the moment passed, and we turned back to staring at the mountains, seeking solace in the rocks and rills. From where we'd perched, I could just make out the pitch of my cabin roof, and right next to it, Justin's.

"What do you know about Justin?" I asked.

"Everything."

"Really?"

A quick grin, reminiscent of the old JJ, flashed across his face. "Just kidding. Uh … I know that he's investing a lot of money—like more than anyone else—in a boys' summer camp that may or may not fail."

"So did you."

"Right. He's crazy."

I couldn't disagree.

"His grandfather died two-and-a-half weeks ago. He has a work ethic unlike anything I've ever seen and no family to speak of."

"His grandpa died?" I asked with a pang of compassion. "Really?"

"Yep."

"Where are his parents?"

JJ shrugged. "Dunno. Said he hardly knew them."

"Did his grandfather raise him?"

"Yeah. He came back from the funeral the same day you returned." He leaned back on his palms. His shoulders eased, and the tension in his face faded. "He had to stay for a little while, take care of some things on the estate."

"Estate?"

"Yeah. His family's loaded. Lives in this big mansion in California. He's old money, I guess."

"I had no idea."

"Me neither at first," JJ said, wiping his hands on his pants. "He's low key like that. He prefers being on his own. Kind of a wanderer. He invested in Adventura because then he could live in the mountains." He paused. "Why do you ask? You gonna break up with Nathan and go for Justin?"

I played it cool, remembering anew that my brothers didn't have all the information. "Mostly curious. I can't get a read on him."

"He's a good guy."

"Hmm."

"How's Nathan?"

"Good," I murmured, feeling the weight of his steady gaze. "Just got a promotion. Do you ever miss Stacey?"

JJ didn't seem as surprised by the question—or rapid change of subject —as I had expected.

"Yeah," he said. "I think so. But it's hard to say. It's been a long time since we broke up." He paused, as if mentally tallying the time. "Four years?"

"Is it *her* you miss?"

He hesitated. "I don't know. I miss knowing someone would be there at the end of the day. Sometimes I get lonely, and I miss her companionship then. But I don't miss the lies and twists and cliffs of our time together. What about you?"

"Me? What about me?"

"Are you happy with Nathan?"

I looked away. "It's complicated."

"You broke up, didn't you?"

My gaze snapped back to his.

"What?"

He ran his tongue over his teeth and grinned. "Don't try to hide it, Meg. I can read you like a book."

I harrumphed, and my shoulders slouched.

"*Cannot.* What gave it away?"

"Coming here." He crossed one ankle over the other. "It seemed like you were running away from something, the way you called and said you wanted the job but wouldn't go into details . You haven't mentioned Nathan once, either. It's not hard to figure out."

"Why didn't you say anything before?"

He shrugged. "Figured you'd tell me when you were ready."

I leaned into him. He wrapped an arm around my shoulder and pulled me close. I'd missed his warm, calming touch. The shriveled part of my heart that had once belonged to Nathan let out a big sigh. It didn't crinkle so much anymore.

"Thanks," I whispered. My appreciation encompassed so much, and I hoped he could sense it. He squeezed me tighter.

"You don't have to hide anything from us, Megara," he said against my hair.

"Thanks," I said, closing my eyes. "For this climb. I needed it."

He squeezed my shoulders.

"Anytime, sister. Anytime."

8

HEAR ME ROAR

A warbling bird outside my cabin ushered in the second week of camp after a luxurious, lazy weekend at the waterfront with JJ and Mark. Forty campers raced through Adventura, smelling like sunscreen and sweat.

Tuesday afternoon, Mark burst into the kitchen from the dining hall, his face streaked with sweat and dirt. His radio squawked.

"I've already talked to Troy," he said into the speaker. "Possible heat exhaustion. Nothing too serious yet. He's got the kid in medical now, and we're monitoring. Over and out."

He tossed both the radio and the clipboard on the island, then dropped to the floor and sprawled, spread eagle, with a groan.

"Oh, man." He threw an arm over his eyes. "What was I thinking? Why did I start a summer camp? Some kid just threw up on JJ at the climbing wall. Another kid won't drink anything but Sprite. He's dehydrated with possible heat exhaustion. And Sione found some kid in the biffy smoking a cigar he stole from his dad."

I grimaced. No matter how far away I went, I didn't miss the vomit side of nursing. Trying to figure out how much chili and corn bread to make for dinner seemed easy in comparison to Mark's ever-evolving job.

"Yikes," I said.

"There's so much to do," Mark said, rubbing his forehead. "I'm not sure we'll get it all done before skit night. Oh, this tile floor feels so cold." He shivered in delight. "It's amazing. I think I'll take a nap."

I whirled around.

"Did you say there's a lot to do? Do you need help with something? I'm free for the next hour."

Mark popped one eye open, then sat up and leaned on one elbow. "Seriously?"

"Yes! Anything to get out of the kitchen."

I grabbed the Clipboard of Power and swung it toward me. As usual, a grid of the day sat on top of a stack of papers. On the left, he'd scrawled a list of chores. I ran my finger along it, then stopped at the last one and tapped on it.

"That. I'll do that."

He climbed to his feet, peering at my choice. "You want to chop wood for the bonfire tonight?"

"Yep."

"Have at it, little blister. Better you than me. The ax is in the storage shed behind the main office. The wood's back there too. Don't forget gloves. You don't want to *have* a blister and *be* a blister."

He departed, guffawing at his own joke.

~

WITH THE HIGH SUN OVERHEAD, I changed into a pair of workout clothes, braided my hair, and headed for the woodpile.

Fifteen minutes later, I hefted the axe in my hands. Seemed lighter than I'd expected. Two chips had broken out of the curve of the blade, which didn't appear all that sharp. Probably wouldn't make a difference. Chopping wood was more about muscle power than blade precision.

I wrangled my first casualty onto a nearby stump with hack marks, then grabbed the ax. After a few practice swings, I took my first shot. The ax embedded itself halfway through the log. I lifted it and slammed it back down. The ax head slipped cleanly through. Three pieces of wood clattered to the ground. I tossed the logs into a nearby wheelbarrow and lugged the next victim over.

No denying it—slamming an axe into something felt *awesome*.

For the next twenty minutes, the physical jolt of swinging the ax and feeling it bite the logs, cleaving them into smaller chunks, sang through my arms. I let fly, enjoying the movement of my muscles and the satisfying *thwack* of the axe.

Just as my arms began to tremble, the ax embedded itself partway into a log. I gripped the handle close to the head and tried to pump it loose. Nothing. I slammed the log onto the stump to force the axe through, but it didn't budge.

For ten minutes, I wrestled the wooden beast in every possible position. Breathless, I leaned back, wiping sweat off my forehead.

"You gotta … be kidding," I muttered. No inanimate object would defeat me.

Shavings of wood, perfect for kindling, scattered the ground. I reached down to gather them and give my weary arms a rest. Just as I collected a neat handful, a splinter slid into my nail bed with finite, precise agony. I jerked my hand back.

"Ow!"

Just seeing the splinter embedded in my nail made my toes curl. My fingertips blanched white from squeezing them into my palm. I rolled my lips together to keep from screaming.

"Hey, Meg. Nasty splinter?" a voice called from the trees. Justin stepped into view wearing a holey pair of pants flecked with wood stain, his face and neck sweaty. My hair had started to fall out of the braid in frizzing strands, pasting itself to the side of my neck as I worked. Every tiny bone in my hands seemed to tremble, radiating agony into my shoulders. Sweat dripped off my face and forearms.

Of course, I thought with cynical amusement. You've seen my underwear. Why not see me scream like a banshee?

"Yep," I gasped. "Just a little one."

Panting from the pain, I turned my back to him. Did I remove the splinter in the safety of my cabin where I could scream into my pillow, or have Troy do it at medical? Something about stalking to the medical cabin seemed humiliating. No. I had to do this on my own. Or with Justin present, as he didn't seem inclined to leave.

He motioned to my hand with a nod.

"You, uh, need some help?"

"Nope. Got it."

He didn't move, so I reached down and plucked the splinter out as if it happened every day. My nostrils flared as the wood slid free. It hurt almost as much coming out as it had going in. The nail pulsed, but soon the strength of the pain faded.

"Burns, doesn't it?" he asked, grinning.

My nostrils flared. "Yep."

He studied me, then motioned to the half-finished log with a nod. "Need some help?"

"Nope." I snatched at the embedded axe. "Got it, thanks."

"Looks like it's stuck."

"Nope. It's good."

Justin shoved his hands into his pockets and leaned back on his heels with a smirk as if to say *show me what you got.*

Ignoring him, I clutched the ax handle in my trembling hands and pulled in a deep breath. I *would* win. This knotted, stingy piece of wood would not embarrass me in front of Justin, of all people. With patience, I finally worked the ax head free, stepped back, and set my teeth.

All right, Megan, I thought. Give your anger wings.

With Nathan's face in the back of my mind, I let out a guttural, warrior-like call and circled the ax down, driving it deep into the wood. Using that momentum, I lifted the ax, log and all, and slammed it back down. Once. Twice. Three times. On the fourth slam, I gathered the last of my reserves.

I will win. I tightened my grip. I will win.

With one last, mighty swing, the axe broke through. Two pieces of knotty pine fell to the ground with dull thuds. My shoulders burned like a magma flow.

Justin stared, eyes wide.

"Do you need anything?" I asked, fiercely proud of myself.

A slow grin spread across his face. He started to laugh. Low, at first, like thunder. It gained volume in his belly and then rolled out in the deepest laugh I had ever heard.

The corners of my mouth twitched.

"You should see yourself." He wiped the corner of his eye. "Oh, Meg. You should see yourself. Good work. Good. Work."

He turned away, still chuckling.

"I am woman." I drove the axe into the stump. "Hear me roar."

THE HOT, soapy dishwater turned my fingertips into raisins the next morning. My wounded fingernail stung for the first five minutes of washing and then went numb.

Behind me, the dull thud of footsteps echoed through the dining hall. The kitchen door swung open and closed again. I set the last dish on a towel to air dry and wiped my hands off on my apron. When I turned around, no one was there.

Odd.

I reached behind me and undid my apron strings, tossing the apron onto a hook on the wall. The familiar hint of vetiver lingered in the air. I pulled a paper calendar off the fridge and studied it. Sandwiches for lunch. Again.

Feeling a bit more adventurous than usual, I reached for Grandma's recipe book. As I skimmed the entries, my phone rang from the top of the fridge. I answered while perusing a Naked Black Forest Cake recipe.

"This is Megan," I said into the phone.

Baker's chocolate? I thought, staring at the list. How is that different from regular chocolate?

"Megan Bailey," said a low, feminine voice. "This is Jodie Renner from EveryHealth Corporation."

My heart leaped into my throat. I slammed the book shut.

"Jodie the nurse recruiter?"

"Yes. I hope you don't mind, but I pulled your phone number from our old employment records."

"Oh, no. I don't mind."

"I thought this would be easier than email. Can you talk?"

I darted to the swinging door and peered into the dining hall. Empty. Only the fans rotated overhead. Outside, campers and counselors chattered around each other. The pantry door was closed. I let out a long breath and stood by the back door, just in case someone strolled up.

"Sure. What's up?"

"I'm happy to hear that you're interested in a job with EveryHealth Corporation. Karen and I have been friends for years. She speaks very highly of you."

"Thank you."

"My job as nurse recruiter is to find the right person for the right job. EveryHealth is committed to their patients—we only hire the best. Your resume is impressive, Megan. I think we can find a position for you."

"That's good to hear. I'm mostly interested in flight nursing."

"Ah, yes. I spoke with Blake at West End a few days ago," Jodie said. "He was pretty upset that he couldn't hire you onto their flight team. If you're still interested in a flight-nurse position, I think I can help you out."

Jodie's slightly husky voice moved like a stream of chocolate—soothing, with an occasional ripple. The smooth edges of her words carried a Spanish accent.

"Yes!" I cried and then cleared my throat. "Uh, sorry. I mean—yes. I would love to find a flight-nurse position. But I'm currently working at my brothers' summer camp. I won't be available to work for at least six weeks."

"Hmm..." She tutted under her breath. "That could complicate things."

My heart fell into my stomach like a stone.

"Oh?"

"Well, you see, getting you a flight position can be tricky. It's all about timing. But let's not worry about that until we have to. Could you leave the summer camp if I find something for you?"

I leaned back against the fridge, one arm folded across my middle. The warm summer air had started to turn tacky. Would I leave Adventura? I needed a job eventually. The little issue of the credit card bill popped back into my mind. I bit my bottom lip.

"I don't know if I could leave the camp, to be honest. My brother had a hard time finding anyone to do this job."

"Are you a nurse there?"

"No. I cook for the staff."

"Ah, yes. Well, that's easily replaceable, isn't it?"

I hesitated, unsure of what to say. Cooking hadn't been *easy*, but it hadn't been rocket science either. Surely someone else could do it.

"Maybe?"

"Well, something to think about. We'll just move forward and see what we find. If I can't find you a flight-nurse position, how do you feel about another Intensive Care Unit?"

My mind strayed to my mortgage, car payment, and the credit card bill burning a hole in my backpack. A generous sign-on bonus could almost cover the credit card—18% interest included. Jodie's voice drew me out of my thoughts.

"I don't see a Respiratory ICU on your resume," Jodie continued. "Maybe we can find you something there?"

"Sure. I'd like that. Uh, I do have a question. Are there any hospitals offering a sign-on bonus?"

"Sign-on bonus? Some do. Not many. I can usually get you relocation. Is a sign-on bonus a deal-breaker for you?"

"No," I said quickly. "Uh, mostly curious."

"Oh, shoot." She let out a long breath. The sound of someone speaking in the background came through the earpiece. "Listen, Megan, I just had someone show up in my office. Can I call you again? I want to get to know you more so I can fit you into the best slot."

"Yes, of course."

"I'm so sorry."

"No problem."

"I'll keep my eyes open, and we'll talk soon. Bye."

Once the conversation ended, I shoved my phone into my pocket and crossed my arms. What if Jodie *did* find a flight position for me? Would I take it? The ring of my promise to JJ echoed in my head.

You always have me.

Until the perfect job comes along, I imagined myself tacking on. A pit grew in the bottom of my stomach. I drove a hand through my hair with an agitated intake of breath. No reason to worry about that yet. Who knew what she'd find? Having Jodie on the search made me feel better. At least I had career cogs moving again. A squeak near the pantry startled me. I whipped around and saw the pantry door move a millimeter.

"Hello?"

It opened an inch. A pair of blue eyes peered out of the crack in the door. Justin waved at me with a sheepish grin on his face. "Just me."

I stacked my hands on my hips.

"Were you spying on me?"

"No!" He held up both hands in a gesture of surrender. "I swear. I just came into the pantry for quiet while I figured out how to fix a storage shed. It's chaos out there, and I can't think in chaos."

He held up a piece of paper with writing on it as proof. My skin frosted into a sheet of ice. He'd been in the pantry the whole time? I shuffled forward a tentative step.

"What did you hear?"

His lips parted. "I swear, Megan, I wasn't trying to spy on you. Just ... consider me deaf. I didn't hear anything."

"But you did."

"Yeah." He readjusted his ball cap. "Yeah, I did hear a few things."

"Like how I'm looking for a job."

He winced. "Yeah."

And how I might have to leave early if I find another position. The unspoken words rotated in the back of my mind like a squeaky wheel. I could barely meet his eyes when I said, "They were making cutbacks. I was the least senior nurse on the floor and got the boot."

"Sorry, Meg. That's tough."

"Work is very important in my family," I said, even though I could see in his eyes that he didn't need an explanation. My shoulders crept higher and higher. "Mark has Adventura, and Mom's a flight-nurse. Dad has been sheriff in Beaumont for ... forever."

"Except for JJ." Justin's dimple made a brief appearance. "Who has never had an official job before Adventura."

Most recently, JJ had lived out of a crappy van he bought from some hippies while he attempted to free climb El Capitan. Before that, he had lived to climb, earning money from races, climbing sponsorships, and guided climbs. He'd never had a true boss. Even now, one could hardly call Mark a *boss*.

A fleeting grin surprised me. "Yes. Except for JJ."

His expression sobered.

"Would you leave?"

My heart pounded. "I don't know. It's just that I ... if I get ... it's complicated. And there's no telling whether she'll even find a flight-nurse position for me. I'll cross that bridge if it comes up."

Justin relaxed into a smile. "Well, next time I have a pantry meeting, I'll schedule it with you."

The teasing glint in his eyes smoothed out my final ruffle. He didn't seem to be horrified by my situation. I smiled. "Thanks."

"Good luck with the job search, Meg. Any hospital would be lucky to have you." He stepped onto the porch and said over his shoulder, "And I hope you don't have to leave early."

Things That Smell Better Than Nathan

- *Not Mark's breath.*
- *Morning.*
- *Wet pine needles.*
- *Campfire.*
- ~~*Skunkweed.*~~
- *Fresh dirt by the creek.*
- *Pink wildflowers.*
- *The sun. On everything.*
- *My soggy tennis shoes.*
- *Vetiver.*

9

NOT YOUR FIGHT

Thursday afternoon, I parked the truck in the heart of Beaumont, a sweet little mountain town twenty minutes outside Jackson City. Dad had been working here since I started elementary school. I'd grown up not far away, right in between Beaumont and the outskirts of Jackson City. Adventura lay only an hour west of Dad's office.

An old-time ice cream store flanked a touristy shop, where two teenagers dressed in feather boas and extravagant hats posed for a tin-type photo. In the background, kids squealed from a wagon pulled by horses as they rode down Main Street. I cut across the road and hurried up the steps of the Sheriff's Department in a pair of jeans and flip-flops.

Rhonda, a pale-faced woman with bright pink lipstick and two chins, sat behind a desk. Her mouth wagged open as I stepped inside the cool, air-conditioned building. It sent chills up my hot skin.

"Oh. Mah. Gawsh. That can't be Maygun Bailey!" she cried, standing up. "Come give Rhonda a hug! I haven't seen you in years."

"Hello, Rhonda," I said stepping into her warm embrace. Her thick arms wrapped around me like a steel trap. She pulled away, gripping me by the arm. Sweat dotted her upper lip.

"What's a big-time nurse like you doing in a place like this?"

"Just here to see my dad." I glanced behind her. "Is he in? I thought I saw his truck outside."

She motioned behind her with a jerk of her head. "He's back there. Just filling out some paperwork from an attempted robbery last night."

"Did he get them?"

Rhonda grinned. "You bet he did. Your Daddy is thuh best."

"Hey!" a gruff voice called from the back. "What kind of riff-raff just walked in my door?"

A tall, imposing figure in wranglers and cowboy boots stepped into the office doorway, filling it with his frame. He set his hands on his hips, glaring at me through hazel eyes.

"Hey there, old man."

"Well, hello there, Miss Bailey," he said in the familiar burr that I knew deep in my bones. He spread out his long arms. "Well? What's taking you so long?"

I rushed over and threw myself at him.

A gentle, quiet laugh rolled through his chest when I pressed the shell of my ear to it, squeezing his ribcage with my arms. He smelled like Old Spice and gunpowder. Strands of salt-and-pepper hair fanned above his ears, highlighting the mellow hues of his eyes. Age seemed to have caught up with him, making his lips thinner, his crow's feet deep as canals. Though still lean and strong, his shoulders bowed as if he carried the invisible burden of time.

"What are you doing here?" he asked, pulling away. "Thought you weren't coming to see me until next week."

"Well, I flew back home for one of Rudy's hamburgers and was tired of waiting for it," I said. "No one makes them like Rudy."

A hint of a smile crossed his lips.

"C'mon." He reached behind him and grabbed his cowboy hat from a nail inside his office. A corkboard filled with pictures of fish hung on the wall next to it. "Let's go out to lunch. Rhonda, call me if you need anything."

Rhonda rolled her eyes. "You never answer."

He winked at me.

"You know where to find me if you need me. Let's go, Megan. I can hear your stomach from here."

Rudy's Diner, a kitschy place with high wooden booths and rustic decorations, buzzed with tourists and locals. The sizzle of the grill and the heady scent of French fries drifted through the restaurant, making my empty stomach growl. A man behind the bar spotted Dad and waved us ahead of the line and into a booth at the back. Dad held up two fingers.

"With everything," he called over the din. The man gave him a thumbs-up.

"You're a celebrity now?" I asked.

A sheepish grin flashed across his face. "I let him out of a parking ticket last week." He set his hat on the bench while I laughed. "Listen, Meg, I'm sorry that I haven't come to see you yet," he said. "Work has been busy."

"I get it."

He grunted. A circle of matted hair ran around his head from his hat. He ran a hand through it, mussing it like Mark's. It fell back into place.

"So, what's going on with you?" I asked. "How's Beaumont?"

"Fine."

"Anything exciting?"

He shook his head. Dad had never been a man of many words. Want to pay off my credit card debt? I thought of sliding in. Or just loan me a couple hundred bucks to keep the sharks at bay until I have a job?

Unemployment never felt so humbling.

"Are you going to come try out Adventura's rifle range with me?" I asked instead, sipping a glass of water that a waitress brought over. Breaking into my debt without incurring the wrath of Dad would require some finesse. "Gary brought a couple of rifles to try on the weekend."

"I could do that." He leaned back in the chair, studying me with narrowed eyes. "Enough about me. I'm boring. I want to hear about you. You gonna marry that Nolan guy?"

"Nathan."

He rolled his eyes.

"Seems unlikely," I said.

"Huh."

Unable to bear the cordial small talk, I leaned forward. "What's going on with you and Mom?"

I expected a flinty expression brimming with irritation, but nothing happened. His eyes closed, as if he'd been waiting for my outburst. He scrubbed a hand over his cheeks, which needed a shave. Music from an old jukebox switched to a Hank Williams song, strumming just below the cacophony of voices.

"That's our business, not yours," he said softly. "Nothing you kids need to worry about."

"My family. My business."

He picked up a roll of utensils and flipped them from end to end with a rhythmic *thunk* on the table. In the silence, a waitress brought two plates each loaded with a greasy hamburger, pickles, and golden fries. She left. Neither of us made a move toward them.

"Things are different, kid," Dad said, his voice low. "Ever since all of you left, it hasn't been the same. The house is quiet. Empty. There's not as much to do at home. Things between your mom and I … shifted."

"How?"

He scowled. "I don't know. It's different. Your mom has work, so I go fishing. She's gone for days at a time, and I started working odd shifts."

The hair on the back of my neck stood up. That didn't sound right.

"Odd shifts? But you always work days."

"That was before your mom left for work all the time." He shrugged. "It's easier to work or hunt or fish while she's gone than just sit at home alone. But then we were both gone all the time. Without you kids there … it just … it's *different*."

A hole opened up in my heart, expanding through my chest. It would swallow me up soon. Disbelief pervaded my thoughts. My parents had always been madly in love … hadn't they? Frequent dates. Passionate kisses. Bouquets of wild irises for no reason. The memory of those flowers filled my nose with their distinct scent.

"So, she started working, and you drifted apart?"

"Yeah. It's like … I stopped mattering to her." He rambled off into another grumble I didn't try to translate.

"What about counseling?"

"Just started."

"And?"

"Too soon to tell."

"Dad, give me something here."

"No. This is *our* business."

We stared hard at each other. The pain in his eyes made my own seem pale in comparison. I relented first. "Fine. I'll stop asking about your business. Can you just tell me whether you think things are salvageable?"

He looked away, and though he promised nothing, his silence at least meant he was thinking about it.

"Nothing's impossible, Meg. But I just ... I just don't see how we can repair something that's been in the making for so many years. We need a little more time, I think."

"Do you ever see each other anymore?" I asked.

He picked at a fry. "Not really."

"Because..."

"It's too hard."

"To see her?"

"Yes."

I held my breath, hardly daring to voice my worst fear. "Did something happen?" My voice croaked. "I mean, did she cheat? Did *you* cheat?"

Just saying the words filled my mouth with a metallic taste. He grabbed one of his pickles and threw it at me. It hit my face with a splat.

"What was that for?" I cried, peeling it off. Ketchup and mustard dripped down my cheek. I wiped it away with my fingers.

"You deserved it!" The hurt in his eyes cut right through me. "How could you even say that?"

"Well, you haven't said what's going on. What am I supposed to think?"

"It's not your business!"

"Fine," I said, holding my hands up. "You're right. I'm sorry. I shouldn't have jumped to conclusions."

He relaxed. "You really want to know why we aren't talking and barely see each other?"

"Yes. I do."

"We fell out of love, Megan. That's what happened." He pounded the table with every word. "It's. That. Simple. It happened slow, over the years. We forgot to take care of each other and just took care of ourselves. We drifted apart."

Tears filled my eyes. I tried to swallow them back, but they brimmed like hot springs. Betrayal simmered hot and humid under my skin. Why didn't they take care of each other? What did marriage mean if not *that*?

"Fine. You fell out of love. You can get it back."

His jaw tightened. "That's what we're trying to figure out."

Betrayal turned to pain, filling my chest with fire and venom and darkness. I couldn't stop it.

"JJ knows something is going on, and he's frustrated that no one will say anything. Mark is ignoring it, probably because he doesn't want it to be real, and I'm so confused I can't sleep at night."

"What do you want me to do, Meg?" he asked, spreading his hands. "What do you want?"

"I want you to fix this! I want you to be honest with us."

"I can't do that on my own."

"Yes, you can. Talk to Mom. Spend time in the same room. Come visit us at Adventura. *Fight*, for heaven's sake!"

He leaned back, his voice vibrating. "Let this go. It's not your fight."

"But I can't! Dad, I'm scared."

"It's not as easy as talking to your mom. If it were that simple, I would have done it long ago."

"Why isn't it that simple?"

"Because I've already tried."

"Try harder! You can't throw this away. It's more than just you two."

"I did try!" he yelled, slamming his palms on the table. "I tried. I tried, Megan. But she's not sure she wants me back. That's why. Are you happy now? After thirty years of marriage, she doesn't want me!"

He balled up his napkin and threw it on the table. With two moves, he grabbed his hat, threw a twenty on the table, and disappeared into the stunned crowd. *Move,* I told my frozen muscles. *Follow him. Move!*

They didn't respond.

Immobilized, I watched him go. A gamut of emotions flooded me. Terror. Uncertainty. Confusion. Regret. I shouldn't have put everything on his shoulders. But ... how could they just fall out of love? How could he let that happen? Why didn't Mom know if she wanted him anymore?

I closed my eyes and sank further into the cushion.

How long had my family been falling apart, and why was I just noticing it now?

~

Operation Reignite My Parents: *Mission Brainstorming*

- *~~Call Mom about conversation with Dad.~~*
- *Reminisce.*
- *Watch Parent Trap for inspiration.*
- *Buy them a puppy.*
- *~~Move back home.~~*
- *Tell JJ?*
- *Send Mom flowers from Dad.*
- *Send Dad takeout Chinese from Mom.*
- *Set the house on fire.*
- *Shave my head and tell them I need counseling. Then drag them to it. Then leave them with counselor.*
- *~~Do nothing.~~*
- *Go on a trail run with Mom.*
- *Try to believe that love is worth it.*
- *Watch Fight Club. (Move to 'Things That Are Crazier Than My Crazy' List)*
- *~~Eat something sugary.~~*

10

SINKING

Friday morning, I woke with the first beams of sunrise.

After sliding in and out of vague dreams, I stopped fighting for sleep that wouldn't come. I slipped from my bag and into the crisp air. When I ventured out of my cabin in long sleeves and my hair in a braid, no life stirred. For now, I had Adventura to myself.

Steam drifted off the lake. I shivered in my shorts as I padded down the gravel path to the waterfront. The loose rock shifted underneath my sandals while I walked, my mind as cloudy as the fog clinging to the water. I continued past the shallow buoys and stopped at the end of the U-shaped pier. Nothing disturbed the water except for glimmers of foraging fish.

By the time I grabbed a paddle board, set it in the shallows, and stepped on top, rays of sunshine pierced the water. The wisps retreated, as if they couldn't bear the light. I sat on the board and paddled to the middle of the lake. My feet dangled off the edge in the cool water. Goosebumps covered my skin, but I pulled my sleeves over my hands and kept going.

The quiet licks of water on the board soothed my static-filled thoughts. I concentrated on the way the oar sank into the lake instead of thinking about Dad not answering my repeated phone calls. I wondered if he'd listened to my apologetic voicemails. Rhonda had hesitated when I asked her why he wouldn't talk to me, and an emptiness rang through my chest.

I shouldn't have pushed so hard. But the terror of losing my parents' marriage pushed me to desperation. Dad would only brood for a day or two, work through it, and call me—he always did. But I still felt a little lost.

To make matters worse, I still had no money and no courage to ask him for any.

Ripples expanded around the oar as I dipped it in the water. Every touch of the lake sent ever-widening rings into the distance until they faded. I stared at them and felt shaken when they disappeared.

A vague sound drew my gaze to the right. Out of the mist came the swing of a powerful arm. I drew my paddle in when Justin's head bobbed above the lake in a silent breath and disappeared into another stroke. He moved swiftly and quietly, like a crocodile. I stared, transfixed by the play of muscle as his arms blazed through the water.

He stopped a few feet short of my board. Water streamed down his face even after he wiped it off, shaking the loose droplets free. His hair twisted into a loop on top of his head.

"Hey." He blew the excess water from his lips in a soft raspberry. "Aren't you supposed to stand up on these things?"

"I like to set my own trends."

"Trailblazer."

"More like lazy. Standing requires more energy than I have this early." I tipped to the side, peering into the murky depths. "Besides, I don't really want to get wet. It takes way too long to warm back up."

"Chicken."

"Nah. I just don't feel like making hot chocolate."

The teasing glint in his eye faded. "What are you doing out here so early, anyway?" he asked.

"Couldn't sleep. Do you swim out here often?"

"Every morning."

I leaned forward. "Really?"

Had I missed so many opportunities to see him shirtless? If the sculpted shoulders and arms I was catching glimpses of while he treaded water bore any similarity to the rest of him, I'd come every morning.

With binoculars.

"Every morning. I grew up on the ocean. This helps the homesickness."

"I didn't know that."

"Do you like to swim?"

"Sure." I shrugged. "I don't do it much, but I *can* swim. I'm not as fast as JJ, though. He beats me at everything."

Justin nodded to the opposite bank. "Hey, check it out," he said in a soft voice. "We have a visitor."

A dusky shape nosed through the reeds at the edge of the lake. A young male moose—his antlers weren't quite impressive yet—stepped out of the fog. I held my breath. Such a beautiful, wild world up here. Always surprising me.

"He's huge," I murmured.

"Not as big as the bull that I've seen every now and then. This guy comes out here most mornings."

"Has he ever bothered you?"

"Nah. I stay away."

"Good plan."

I looked to the opposite bank, expecting to see another dark figure, albeit much smaller, haunting the lake.

"Where's Atticus?" I asked.

"Probably cuddling with JJ. They bonded when I went home."

"JJ loves his own kind," I said. Justin tilted his head back and laughed, giving me a glimpse of his strong neck as the water lapped around it. I turned away. Wildlife was far less intimate than the ring of a farmer's tan around his biceps.

"So," Justin said. "Everything all right? You seemed upset when you got back yesterday."

A blush crept across my cheeks.

"Oh, yeah. Sorry about that whole lunch fiasco."

While I'd been fighting with Dad, the oven had stopped working for no discernible reason. The lasagnas I'd left cooking came out half-frozen in the middle and slushy on the edges when Mark retrieved them at noon. An hour after lunch, the oven flipped back on, which left the kitchen broiling hot the rest of the evening.

Justin's dimple made a quick appearance. "Eh. Nothing anyone could have done about that. They brought the microwave in. Turned out fine."

"My parents are having a hard time," I said, running my finger along the edge of the paddle board. The rough texture felt as stubbled as my thoughts. "I got in a fight with my dad yesterday. That's probably why I looked upset."

"Anything serious?"

I hesitated. "I don't know."

"You want to talk about it?"

"Uh ... do you want me to talk about it?" I asked, eyes narrowing.

He shrugged. "If you want to."

"Can you tread water for hours? Turns out my parents have layers of hidden dysfunction I didn't know about."

"Give me the short version."

I bit the inside of my cheek, unsure of how to wrap it all up in a neat little box that didn't look as hideous as it felt. The water caressed my knee, grounding me back into the moment. How could I explain my disorientation and uncertainty?

"I guess it's simpler than I made it out to be," I said, thinking it over. "They fell out of love."

He winced. "Ouch."

"Doesn't it sound terrible?"

"You'd almost prefer to hear that one of them was addicted to gambling, or they had a lot of debt, or something like that."

I threw my hands in the air. "Yes! Because those things are at least tangible, right? I mean, addictions can be worked on. Debt can be consolidated. But falling out of love?" My hand fell back to my lap. "How do you even fix that?"

"*You* don't. It's up to them."

"What if they don't fix it?"

The confidence in his gaze disarmed me. "Then they don't. And it's going to suck for a while."

Tears threatened again at the back of my throat. I ran my fingers through the water on the paddle board. I hadn't let myself go to that place yet. I cleared my throat.

"Sounds like you have some experience," I said.

"I do."

I stared at him. "Oh. Really?"

"My parents divorced when I was seven. Used me as a pawn for a year or two until my grandpa stepped in. He raised me."

My mouth parted. "Oh, wow. I'm so sorry. I had no idea."

He shrugged. "It is what it is. And yes, it sucked. But I couldn't do anything to save what didn't want to be saved. I thought it was up to me, that year when I bounced back and forth between them. But it's not. Movies like *The Parent Trap*? They're just not that likely."

The helpless, lost feeling returned but not with as much power. Justin had turned out fine, and he didn't have *any* parents. Mine still loved me. Maybe my life wasn't as dark as I made it out to be.

"So," I said, sucking in a deep breath. "What do I do?"

"What do you think you should do?"

I thought it over. "I'm not sure. Try to get them to talk?"

"Or you could leave them to it."

"Maybe stage an intervention?"

He coughed into a fist. "Or do nothing."

"Or," I concluded with a slump of my shoulders. My eyes strayed to the moose, who plodded through the knee-high water, dragging moss as he went. "I could do nothing. Let them sink or swim."

"They'll swim," he said. "Don't worry. There's one more option, you know."

"What is it?"

"You make me a cake."

I reared back. "What?"

He nodded. "I've been treading water this long without drowning myself. I'll need the calories."

I blinked, momentarily disoriented, then splashed him with my paddle. He dodged the water with a chortle.

"Weak!" he called.

I curved the blade of the paddle and cut it into the water at an angle, spraying him again. He held up a hand, staving off the worst of the splash.

"Don't get involved in a war you can't win," he drawled, shaking loose drops of water out of his eyes.

"I have higher ground."

"But I have tactical advantage."

He planted one hand on the board, grabbed my other arm, and yanked. Although I lunged to the other side, he used his body weight to pull me off. The murky water closed around me in a chilly embrace, cutting off my squeal. When I surfaced, Justin had commandeered both the paddle and the board.

"Hey!" I splashed after him. "That's *my* paddle board! And this water is freaking cold!"

He tossed a jaunty grin over his shoulder and hopped with lithe grace onto the board. "Yeah, but your hair needed a good rinse."

"I just washed it yesterday!"

When I attempted to climb on the board, he pushed me off with the paddle. I grabbed a reed out of the water and threw it at him. He stood without so much as a wobble in his legs and glided away.

"Show off," I called.

"Just putting the paddle board to good use," he said. "And ensuring that we don't get oily, stinky hairs in our breakfast."

"You haven't seen the last of me, Mackleby." I shoved the hair out of my eyes. "I will win!"

"Sink or swim, Meg," he said, without turning around. "Let them decide."

"Yeah," I muttered. "Like it's that easy."

The muscles of his back shifted like a choreographed dance with every stroke of the paddle. With a snort to clear the remnants of water from my nose, I started an easy breaststroke back to shore. Just behind me, the young moose drifted into the trees, nothing more than shadow.

~

Megan,

Sorry about cutting our conversation short a few days ago. Would you like to continue our discussion via video chat? I'd also like to conduct an informal interview. I always prefer working with candidates face-to-face if I can. Not essential, just a preferential quirk of mine. Also, I've found a few job opportunities I'd like to discuss with you.

Wednesday morning would be a convenient time for me. Please let me know if it works for you.

Regards,
Jodie Renner

Lizbeth greeted me with a sleepy wave of her hand when I stepped into the Frolicking Moose on Wednesday. The smell of warm vanilla and pastries washed over me. An old woman haunted the corner, nursing a coffee mug while reading her newspaper.

"Internet?" Lizbeth asked.

"And an iced tea?"

"On it."

I found a chair at the back. The intonation for Skype rang as I pulled the phone out of my pocket. *JRenner* popped up with a video chat request. I sucked in a deep breath and clicked on the icon. Five seconds later, an unfamiliar face filled my screen.

"Megan Bailey," Jodie said, "wonderful to finally see you."

Hair black as a raven fell to her shoulders in a long waterfall, accenting her shadowy eyes and tawny skin. A burgundy silk shirt was buttoned almost to her neck, revealing part of a diamond necklace. Warm cherry wood walls lined the background. She held a pair of black glasses in one hand. A massive diamond ring caught the light in dazzling rays.

"You as well."

She leaned forward. "Let's get right to it, shall we? I have a few questions before we start with specifics."

"Sure."

We launched into the quick back and forth of typical interview questions. How do you deal with stress? What is your five-year plan? What is your ideal job? What would you do in a situation that pitted you against a patient or a doctor?

I forced myself to relax. Still, my nerves felt stretched thin by the end. Jodie had an intensity about her that I hadn't seen since I left the Intensive Care Unit. Suddenly, the carefree, easygoing nature of the staff at Adventura struck me as far more comfortable.

"Very good." She scribbled one last note, then set her pen down. "Thank you for indulging me."

She stared right into the screen with her liquid eyes. Her voice, so melodic and deep, dropped a little.

"So, let's get to the nitty-gritty. I've been looking around, but I don't see anything in a flight department. They tend to have their own rules, as you know. Sometimes it's beyond me to get a candidate in. Sometimes it's not. I had a nibble, but they also went with an internal hire. Also, I haven't found any hospitals offering hiring bonuses. Sorry."

My heart sank.

"Oh. I see."

"That doesn't mean I've given up hope. I'll continue to keep an eye peeled. Are you willing to move?"

Lexie would be gone soon. Bitsy had a new business opening. Rachelle always came up with some plan. I had no job. No real ties to my Midwest home. A new beginning seemed ... seductive. I squared my shoulders.

"Yes. I think I would."

She scrawled on a piece of paper. "Good. That helps. There are a few other hospitals across the country in our corporation that I can look into, so don't give up on a flight position yet. Now, I have a position at a Respiratory ICU across town. You wouldn't have to move. The pay is two dollars more than you made before, with matching 401(k) and better benefits. The position will go fast. Would you like to apply?"

"When does it start?"

Her eyes crisscrossed down a computer screen. "Two weeks."

I swallowed. "Oh. I can't. I'm here at camp."

She frowned, her lips pursed. "I didn't realize that was still in the way. You're planning on staying at the camp all summer, then?"

My mouth turned dry.

"Uh, yes. Unless..."

She allowed my response to trail away. She folded her hands together and let out a long breath.

"I see. Well, let's be honest, Megan. There's no reason for me to look until you're ready. Most of these positions have immediate needs. Perhaps we should speak again when you're closer to coming home?"

A bolt of panic zipped through me.

"Oh, I still want a job!"

"Of course. But we're wasting time if I keep track of current positions. Email me two weeks before you're available. We'll discuss options then. How does that sound?"

I leaned closer to the computer. "Can you keep an eye open for a flight position?"

"Of course. I'll contact you if I find anything. Best of luck at camp, Megan."

The screen went blank.

My mind numbed, uncertain what to feel first. Jodie had a point—why search until I could commit? But not having my career move forward opened a deep chasm in my chest.

My thoughts rotated to Mom and Dad, then Mark and JJ. Dad and JJ had no emotional ties to their jobs. Mark, Mom, and I did. All of us had our own problems. I thought of Nathan for the first time in days, and my spiral deepened. The lack of answers frightened me most.

And the little question of my growing debt lingered in the back of my mind.

The filmy threads of my future seemed to dance in front of me, tantalizing and ethereal. When I reached out, they faded into nothing. Sighing, I stood up. Jodie would keep an eye out for flight-nurse positions. All hope wasn't lost yet. I could still ask Mom for money.

And sort my life out in the meantime.

11

ESCAPING

Riding into Jackson City that weekend sent a thrill through me; I wanted to walk through the heart of downtown and reminisce instead of haunt the same trails that had started to lose their excitement thanks to morning runs with JJ. Mom and I used to shop at the farmers market every weekend in the summer. Smelling the gritty freshness would remind me of happier times.

"Hey there, girl power," Justin said, unlocking the driver's side door of his Jeep. "Get in any more axe fights lately?"

He chuckled at his own joke and slid inside before I could respond.

Gary sat next to me in the back seat. Except for a warm smile, he made no attempt at conversation. Troy and Justin discussed a baseball game they were going to watch at a bar, and I let my thoughts wander.

Going to the farmers market in Jackson City today, I texted Mom. *Can you come with?*

She responded within the minute.

Can't. On a 24-hr shift. Sorry. :(

I thought about my conversation with Dad and shoved my phone deep into my pocket.

"We're leaving at two," Justin said once we'd parked, the lights on his Jeep flashing. "Just meet us at the bar?"

"Yeah. Thanks."

He flashed me a quick grin before turning away, strolling down the street with Gary and Troy. My stomach dropped. Nathan's face fluttered through my mind briefly, but the sight of Justin's adorable dimple edged it out.

I wandered between the stalls in the farmers market, running my fingers over fresh squash and strawberries, laughing with the locals and using cash from Mark to buy sun-ripened veggies. After perusing a stand with Native American jewelry, I left the crowded square to find a coffee shop. Most of the local stores were too touristy for my taste. Comic black-bear knickknacks. Cheesy t-shirts. Photos of wildlife.

Just when I ducked into a coffee shop, my phone vibrated. A picture of Lexie's face filled the screen. I pressed the phone to my ear.

"Hey, Lex. How—"

"He proposed!"

I stopped in the middle of the shop.

"Shut. Up."

"I know!" She squealed. I could picture her jumping up and down, blonde ponytail waving on top of her bed. "I can't belieeeeeve it!"

My mouth worked up and down in disbelief.

"I'm dying," she said. "I'm so excited I'm not even hungry. Can you believe it? There *is* something on this planet that's bigger to me than food."

"Your diamond ring, I'm assuming?"

"*No.*" She snorted. "Okay, well ... maybe. It's so sparkly!"

"Tell me everything!" I said, recovering my wits. "I want the whole story!"

"Well, I certainly didn't call to talk about how I missed three workouts this week. Are you ready for this?"

I lowered myself onto a chair.

"Ready."

"So, I was walking home from work—I know, I know. It's so unlike me to walk to work. But Bitsy's been on an exercise rampage since you left, so if I walk to work she counts the miles as my workout, and I've actually really started to look forward—"

"Lexie..." I growled.

"Story. Right. Anyway, it's nothing big. You know Bradley isn't going to draw attention to himself, and all I ever want is food. I was just getting dressed to go to a yoga class with Bitsy when the doorbell rang. I answered it wearing my favorite yoga pants, I might add, and feeling very svelte and thinnerized by the black material. Bradley was standing there on the porch."

"Did you know he was coming?"

"No."

"Did you scream?"

"Well, yes, but only because he was holding a box of those gourmet cupcakes from the new bakery. Okay, it wasn't a scream, per se. More of a hungry bellow. Don't get me wrong, I was happy to see him. But *really* happy to see those cupcakes."

"Did he get the Oreo Lover's Delight?"

"Did he ever." She sighed. "Like half a dozen. So, anyway, I opened the box and went right in. I mean, what goes better before a workout than a big pile of cake and frosting?"

"Ideal pre-workout food."

"Moments before I bit into it, I noticed a sparkle on top of the cupcake. It was the ring! I almost swallowed it whole."

"A true disaster."

"He would have had to buy another one because I would not have fished for it. Anyway, at that point, my eyes saw the ring, but my brain didn't register it. So I just stared at it for, like, I don't know, a minute? Which was perfect because then I looked over and Bradley was on one knee."

"Was he nervous?" I asked.

"Trembling. He was wearing those stupid old cargo shorts and a football jersey. The boy needs a fashion intervention. Not that I'm one to talk. I just figured out that kitten heels have nothing to do with cats."

An old woman ambling by shot me a glare when I laughed out loud. The image of Lexie going in for a cupcake while Bradley proposed in grungy, old college clothes made my eyes water. I wiped the tears away with the back of my hand.

"Oh, Lexie. That's wonderful."

"It really is. I never thought I'd get married. I dreamed of it, sure. But to actually get married? Seems pretty wild." She paused. "I'm thinking Bundt cake at the reception. Or cupcakes. Maybe cake pops, but that feels too progressive."

"Does it have to be cake?"

"I'm not going to answer that. I think I'll write Little Debbie about catering options. Nothing would be more appropriate. Can you imagine a pile of cosmic brownies topped with one of those bride-and-grooms? Stahp! I can't think about it anymore. I'm getting all swoony."

"Have you told your mom?"

"She wept. She almost loves Bradley more than me."

"Bitsy?"

"Haven't told her yet." Even through the phone, I could sense Lexie's grimace. "Not sure how that's going to go. I'm going to buy her a green smoothie and tell her after yoga, when she's all zen."

"She'll be happy for you, Lex."

"I know. She just hates change."

"So, what'll happen after you get married?"

"Sex. Definitely sex. Lots of sex. In the dark. And maybe while I'm fully clothed. I have these love handles that I'm a little insecure about. But he's gorgeous, so I want *him* butt naked."

I rolled my eyes. "But what about after the honeymoon? What comes next for you?"

She paused. "Uh ... not sure."

Her hesitation said it all.

"You're going to move, aren't you?" I asked. The heaviness I'd felt when Lexie announced they'd gone ring shopping returned. Of all the best friends I'd lost to the world of marriage, I'd miss Lexie most.

"It, ah, seems likely, yes. Does that upset you?"

I swallowed. *Yes, it upsets me!* But I'd never tell her that.

"No. Not at all! Lexie, you're going to be married. Of course you would move. You and Bradley are going to make cute little babies and live in a house with a fence and—" A lump of emotion built in my throat. "It's going to be wonderful."

She sighed, seeming relieved. "We will have beautiful children. But whenever I get pregnant, I'm going to hold water like a cow."

I chuckled quietly at first, then with increasing volume until both of us were rolling with laughter. Hilarity helped stave off the disorientation. Why hadn't Nathan and I worked out? Was there something wrong with me that fractured all of my relationships?

"Anyway," Lexie said, "I have to go make some phone calls and avoid the four cupcakes waiting for me in the kitchen."

Grateful for some time and space to think, I nodded.

"Yes. Of course. I'm honored to rank above them. Go make your phone calls, bride. And congrats, Lex. You and Bradley are going to be very happy together."

"We better," she muttered. "Or those Oreo cupcakes are going down this hatch for nothing."

~

Bought you a drink at the coffee shop, I texted Mom after finishing at the cafe. *Are you off saving a life?*

Nope! Come see me. I hope it involves chocolate?

Always. See you in the lobby.

Drinks in hand, I slipped into St. John's Medical Hospital in downtown Jackson City. A cheery receptionist greeted me just as Mom stepped off the elevator.

"Great timing," she said, tucking her hair behind her ear. "Just got off the bird a while ago. We had to transport to Idaho."

"Lowlanders again?"

She winked. "Always. C'mon. Let's sit at a table outside."

The sun streamed through a few quaking aspens, warming sections of my t-shirt when we settled onto a bench. The leaves fluttered like green coins on the wind, clattering together in a light applause.

"Hot chocolate over ice." She sighed after a long draw on her straw. "It's a happy thing."

"I would have gotten a bigger size, but I didn't have enough money on my gift card."

"This is perfect and delicious."

Speaking of gift cards, I thought. How about you loan me five hundred dollars?

I chewed on my straw while Mom prattled about her shift. Her tan skin glowed, and her eyes sparkled. She looked like a totally different person than the woman I'd seen two weeks ago. I harbored a careful hope that it had something to do with reconciling with Dad. Maybe their counseling sessions had improved?

"Wish you had been there, Meg." She snapped her fingers. "You would have had that IV the first time."

I leaned back against the bench. "You seem happy, Mom."

She bit her bottom lip. "When I'm at work, I really am. Listen, I should apologize for falling apart on you last time."

"No, it's fine. Listen, Mom, I wanted to talk to—"

"It's just ... it's all so complicated these days." She released a sharp breath, hot and fast. "Why does life get harder? I'm in my fifties. Shouldn't I be settling into grandkids and retirement?"

"Whoa, whoa."

She held up a hand. "Rhetorical, don't worry. I just don't get why life has to complicate itself."

"Good question," I muttered.

Mom glanced down at her fidgeting fingers. "Your father and I met up the other day at the coffee shop to talk outside of counseling."

Any hope of talking about my debts faded. My stomach clenched, bracing for another blow.

Please be good news.

"How'd it go?" I asked. If she noticed my forced nonchalance, she didn't let on.

"Fine. Well ... awkward. And tense. We both had to miss our counseling appointment last week, but we're going to go again this week."

"That's good, right?"

The thread of longing in my tone couldn't be denied.

"I think so," she said with a rueful breath. "We fought for a while, of course. Over something stupid that I can't even remember. I've been able to pick up some extra shifts at work, so that helps a little. If I think too much, I get sad, so I put it in the back of my head and work. Work helps a lot."

"Has it?"

She turned, lips pouting. "What do you mean?"

I scrambled to explain, then realized that *I* didn't even know what I meant. Something lurked just out of reach in my mind, like a dark thought

I couldn't quite latch onto. Mom didn't really seem like she was working. It seemed like she was ... escaping.

"I don't know. Just ignore me."

She slurped her hot chocolate. "Have you seen your dad yet?"

"I visited him a couple of days ago."

"And?"

Her voice elevated a little too far. I moved to sip my iced tea but ended up just playing with the straw. The nausea in my stomach made it difficult to drink.

"Didn't go well."

Her shoulders softened. "Did he get mad?"

"Kind of. But I pushed him into it."

Mom sat back and rolled her eyes. "He has a temper, that's for sure."

"When did you fall out of love with him?" I asked, blithely ignoring her question. "How did it happen?"

Her back stiffened. "He said we fell out of love?"

"Well ... yes, but Mom, I'm not an idiot. It's what I've *observed*."

"Oh."

"Please tell me there's some kind of hope."

She folded her arms across her middle as if chilled despite the hot, dry air. "I don't know, Meg. There's a lot of water under that bridge."

"He said ... that you didn't want him anymore."

"He's right."

I winced, feeling the pain all the way into my bones.

"I don't want him as he is and has been for years now. Cold. Aloof. Indifferent. He refuses to do things with me. Only wants to hunt and fish. If that's who he is, I don't want anything to do with it. Your father isn't the same man I married years ago."

"I see," I said, although I didn't. Not at all.

Of course he isn't, I wanted to say. Thirty years of life separates you from that guy!

Despite her attempt at being brave, pain laced her words. I could feel it rolling off her. I closed my eyes. What did I know about marriage or relationships? All of mine had failed. A gigantic cloud, tufted like marshmallow puff, drifted over the sun, casting a long shadow. I rubbed my arms.

Mom wrapped an arm around me.

"Megan, I'm grateful you have a solid career. Look at the situation I'm in: A marriage turned cold. Facing retirement. A possible..." She swallowed. "A possible divorce at fifty years old. Without my job, I'd have no way to sustain myself."

My heart felt heavy. It all seemed so jumbled and confusing. What if Mom hadn't had such dedication to her job? Or Dad to his hobbies? Was there a way to straddle the necessary and the desired? Had my career aspirations caused my failed relationships? I cleared my throat, not ready to go there.

"So, Lexie's engaged," I said. "Bradley just asked."

Mom's eyes lit up. "Really? That's fantastic! How did it happen?"

I grinned. "With Oreo cupcakes."

"I've got to hear this."

The sun came out from behind the puffy cloud, warming me again. Mom and I dissolved into laughter as I recounted Lexie's near tragedy. The darkness I sensed on the horizon abated. For a few minutes, I could almost forget the issues we were facing. I drank in the freedom. The laughter.

Right then, I was just a daughter, and Mom was just a mom, and nothing else mattered. I tucked the rest away and relished the warmth.

~

Things More Important to Me Than Work

- *JJ*
- *Mark*
- *Mom*
- *Dad*
- *Lexie*
- *Bitsy*
- *Mira*
- *Rachelle*

~

The rest of the weekend passed in a quiet blur of sleeping in and hiking with Mark, JJ, and Justin. My muscles felt loose when I went to bed Sunday night and slipped into a heavy, restful sleep.

Monday rolled in on the heels of the devil. The morning passed in a frenetic rush of breakfast dishes, hash browns, and scrambled eggs. By the time I cleaned up breakfast, I only had an hour before lunch prep. I grabbed the recipe book and leaned against the island, fanning a piece of paper in front of my face.

"Meg," Mark barked through the radio. "Get to the medical office. Now."

"On my way."

Brenden, a counselor, was standing outside the medical office when I jogged over. He pushed his hat so the brim rested on top of his head, allowing a glimpse of his blue eyes and soft blond curls.

"It's Gary," he said. "Something's wrong. I brought him from the rifle range."

Mark sat next to the old ex-infantryman on a cot, one hand on Gary's bent shoulder as Gary retched into a garbage can. My snap into Nurse Megan happened without prompting. I couldn't figure out how many bell peppers to cut up for a stir-fry for ten men, but medical emergencies were my jam.

"Troy's taking care of a kid at the waterfront," Mark said. "I worried this might be your expertise anyway."

I knelt at Gary's side, eyes darting in assessment. Sweaty forehead. Clenched fists. Definitely experiencing some kind of pain. A stethoscope hung off a nail just above the cot. I snatched it and popped the earbuds in.

"Gary? Can you talk?"

He shook his head with a gasp.

"What happened?" I asked Mark. "When? And how long has he been like this?"

"He started vomiting after breakfast," Brenden said from the doorway. "Didn't really stop. I radioed Mark to ask for help. It's like Gary lost all strength. Grabbed his shoulder, said it hurt. Dropped to his knees."

Gary's heart slammed through my stethoscope like a drum. Sweat rolled down the sides of his face in beads.

"Where's the pain, Gary?"

He grabbed at his chest, panting.

"Does it feel like an elephant is sitting on your chest?" I asked. Gary nodded.

"Heart attack?" Mark mouthed.

I shrugged, although my nurse senses tingled. Bounding pulse. Struggling breath. Strange coloring around the lips. I'd seen this almost every day at work. But I wasn't *at* work where I could know for sure. I was stuck in the middle of a summer camp at least an hour from the nearest hospital.

"Gary, take big, deep breaths for me while I take your blood pressure. Mark, help me lay him on his right side. Keep the garbage right below him."

Gary moaned but let us direct him. I stopped taking his blood pressure so he could dry heave. Mark waited, a comforting hand on Gary's shoulder until I deflated the cuff and pulled the stethoscope out of my ears.

"Bad?" Mark asked.

"High."

I ripped the velcro apart. "Call 911. We'll meet them at the highway. Tell them it's a suspected heart attack and to alert St. John's we're coming. Brenden, find Justin. I need him to drive us."

While they dispersed to do my bidding, I scrambled through the cupboards for an aspirin. Gary moaned, eyes screwed shut, hands clenched, and body limp. I sat next to him with a soothing hand on his back.

"We'll take good care of you, Gary."

A few minutes later, Justin pulled up in the truck.

"Ambulance is on their way," Mark said, throwing open the door. "Said it'll take thirty minutes to get to the turnoff."

Justin stepped inside.

"Jeep is ready to go, Meg."

"Load him up," I said, grabbing a spare oxygen tank and the mask next to it. I slid into the backseat with Gary, placing his head on my lap, the oxygen tank between my legs. Justin pulled away from medical with the crunch of gravel under the tires. Adventura disappeared behind us within seconds.

"Slow or fast?" Justin asked, meeting my gaze in the rearview mirror.

Gary moaned.

"Medium. I don't want him bouncing all over the place back here.

But…" My eyes trailed over his moist face and clenched eyes. "Don't take your time, either."

I slipped the regulator onto the oxygen tank and tightened it, then grabbed the attached green key, tacked it on the top, and turned. Oxygen flowed into the mask. I strapped it to Gary's face and murmured to him.

The drive to the highway took longer than usual, even with Justin's well-paced speed. We pulled up right as the flashing lights of the ambulance twirled into sight. A middle-aged woman with blonde hair and a light blue uniform leaped out of the passenger seat. The driver followed.

"Is it just the two of you?" I asked, ducking down to drape one of Gary's arms around my shoulders. Justin took the brunt of his weight as we hobbled him to the gurney. The woman snapped on a pair of gloves while Justin and the driver helped Gary stretch across the gurney.

"Yep," she said. "The name's Wanda. We're looking to hire some others, but the pool is pretty small around here. You don't have a license, do you?"

"I'm a registered nurse."

"Good enough for me. I'm just an EMT. I could use your help."

"You're kidding," I said, following her into the back of the ambulance. The driver shut one door. Wanda shot me a deadpan expression.

"This isn't the city, honey. It's not always perfect around here. We're low-staffed today thanks to a sick call-out, and we do the best we can. You're lucky we have a driver."

"Right. Not kidding."

"I'll follow you into Jackson," Justin said while Wanda secured Gary with the straps. "And I'll text Mark to let him know."

"Thanks."

The driver slammed the second door.

"I haven't placed an IV in a while," Wanda said, a wad of bright pink gum smacking between her teeth. A rubbery tourniquet flopped onto the package next to her. "Certainly not on a black man." She peered at his hand and wrist. "Can't see a damn vein on him."

"You haven't done an IV on a black man?"

"This is Wyoming. You wanna try first?"

I opened my mouth to express my disbelief but shut it again. I'd never ridden in the back of an ambulance before, and I certainly hadn't ever placed an IV in a moving vehicle. What were the odds that Wanda—likely the only EMT in the area—hadn't placed an IV *in a while*? IVs were the lifeblood of ambulance riders.

"Don't get many calls?" I asked, ripping the package open.

She shook her head. "We're volunteers who live in the mountains." Her teeth flashed with a momentary grin. "We don't even call each other."

"Can you switch to your oxygen source?" I asked. "Mask him at ten liters. And do you have an aspirin? Look for sublingual nitroglycerin, too."

"On it."

Prepping Gary's skin for the IV, opening the package, and working with a saline flush turned all my instincts on. My hands worked by pure muscle memory. I fell into the familiar task with confidence.

"All right, Gary," I said, holding onto his right hand. "There's going to be a little pinch."

The needle slid into the vein with ease. I held my breath—I always did—and waited for the flashback of blood. Like a congratulations, it came.

"Got it?" Wanda asked, peering over him. She'd just finished putting a mask over his face and cranking the oxygen up. It fogged when he exhaled. He grimaced, his head rolling to the side.

"Yep. Prep your cardiac monitors. We need to do an EKG on the way in."

She lifted one eyebrow. "Can you read a 12-lead EKG?"

"Yep."

"All right," she drawled. "You're the boss."

When we arrived at St. John's ER, nurses, doctors, phlebotomists, and respiratory therapists swarmed Gary while I reported to the doctor. The events unfolded like a song. Ten minutes after our arrival—a second EKG, a cocktail of medication, and two lab draws later—Gary sped past me on a gurney into the cath lab. Diana, his nurse, moved to my side. She wore her silver hair in a loose bun on top of her head. Her warm brown skin, wide face, and deep umber eyes indicated she had Native American ancestry somewhere. Her stethoscope and name tag jingled when she walked.

"His labs are sky-high so far." She ran her thumb up in the air. "Never seen 'em that high in my life, and I've worked here a long time. I think he'll be all right, though."

Wanda pitched some paperwork to me. I settled into a rolling chair at the nurses' station and filled it out. The smell of rubbing alcohol, the tinkle of a phlebotomy cart, and the overhead voice paging doctors danced through my mind. My stomach clenched. I missed this.

Oh, *how* I missed this.

When I finished charting, Justin stepped through the swinging doors, bringing a hot wind with him. His brow furrowed when he saw me. "Everything okay?"

"No word yet from the cath lab."

"Is that good news?"

I managed a wry smile. "It's better than bad news."

"Where will he go from there?"

"A room on the floor," Diana said, butting in with a smile. "The two of you are welcome to sit in the waiting room. I'll let you know when they have a room number and a time. And thanks for your help, Megan. That's the best report from a bystander I've ever had."

I let out a deep breath and smiled.

"My pleasure, Diana."

12

TESTS

Hours later, Justin gripped the steering wheel of his Jeep in one hand as he navigated away from Jackson City. He ran a hand through his hair.

"So ... that got intense."

We'd waited until Gary's daughter, Mylee, had driven up to stay with him in the hospital. After a successful heart stent in the cath lab—and several months of cardiac rehab—

Gary was expected to make a full recovery.

I blew out a breath that made my hair dance.

"Heart attacks usually are."

We sped down a long stretch of highway toward the canyon. The sun shone through the windshield in long white rays, making the dust motes shimmer in the air. A text message popped up on my phone.

Just heard, Mom said. So proud of you. That's my girl!

I slipped my phone back into my pocket.

"You did awesome, though. Like, no hesitation." Justin sliced a hand through the air. "Just *boom*! Saved his life. I'm way impressed. So now I'm thinking that I should actually make *you* a cake."

He wore his old baseball cap. The muscles along his forearm flexed and relaxed, as if he were tightening and releasing his fist on purpose.

After our little confrontation at the lake, I couldn't stop staring at his arms.

"A lot of people saved his life. The ambulance driver. Wanda. You. The cath lab doctor. It's hardly ever just one person."

Justin lifted an eyebrow. "But you were the main person. You took over at camp when Mark and I wouldn't have known what to do. And let's be honest: Troy probably wouldn't have either. He's great. But young."

"Thanks for following the ambulance," I said, tucking my hands under my thighs. "And bringing me back to Adventura."

"No problem. I've been texting Mark updates. Apparently his lunch tasted so bad that the staff is revolting and asking for you back."

"I doubt that."

His brow furrowed. "Why?"

"Oh, I just haven't been the best lunch lady, I think."

I studied him from the corner of my eye but couldn't get a good read. I'd been serving different variations of sandwiches for weeks now at lunch. No doubt they were about to organize a walk-out. Justin's lips drooped, but he said nothing more.

I closed my eyes, replaying the moments in the ER. The whir of activity. Shouting voices. As the nurse, coordination of the room often fell to me. I loved it. I loved being so integral to the process. Most of all, I loved knowing that Gary lived.

Several minutes had passed before I pulled myself out of my haze. The emotional high of the past several hours had started to fade. I felt like an overcooked noodle. I wanted to nap, dance, scream, and laugh all at the same time.

"Penny for your thoughts," Justin said after a long stretch of silence.

"I miss it." The words flew out of my mouth before I could stop them. "I miss it so much I feel homesick."

"Your job?"

"Yes."

The smooth granite walls of the canyon flashed by. Justin listened while I rambled about how wonderful it felt to be part of a team, to know what I was doing, to feel confident in my decisions. I wasn't sure I made sense, even as the steam died out.

"You belong to a team at Adventura," he said.

I snorted. "A team that's indifferent, at best."

He frowned. "That's not fair. You haven't given us a chance."

My mouth bobbed open and closed for a second. A tinge of defensiveness had crept into his voice. I couldn't help but notice the *us* in his comment.

"The staff doesn't say much," I said.

"You don't either."

My mouth dropped. "Yes, I do!"

He held up a finger. "You never eat with us." A second finger joined the first. "On weekends, you hang out with your brothers. You hardly ever leave the kitchen."

A cold feeling washed down my arms. "I leave the kitchen," I mumbled.

"You've never joined any of the staff game nights or activities, right? Or weekend poker games? Night hikes? Not once that I remember."

I reviewed the past weeks at Adventura with a growing pit in my stomach. The heat of shame accompanied it. I really hadn't made much of an effort, had I? I fell into my thoughts, turning the idea over and over again. The span of silence grew heavy. He alternated staring at the road and staring at me, cutting smooth arcs along the road as we followed the winding river.

"Are you going to leave Adventura?" he asked. His jaw had tightened. I couldn't help but wonder what he thought of me.

"No." I drew my knees up to my chest. "I wouldn't do that to Mark."

He let out a long breath. "Good. That would destroy him, and not just because it would really mess up Adventura."

I stared out the window, catching a glimpse of my reflection. Thoughts of Jodie flickered through my mind, and I wished I could take my words back. Maybe I *would* leave. I thought of Mom outside the hospital, happy in the sunshine of her job but swimming through a failed marriage. My stomach tightened.

No, I decided. *People are more important than jobs.*

~

WITH JUSTIN'S advice ringing in my head the next morning, I stood in the kitchen and stared out at the dining hall. A typical Tuesday morning. The smell of coffee beans circled through the lodge, melting into the saccharine scent of warm syrup. Four towering stacks of pancakes had dwindled into only one short stack. I flipped two onto my plate, shoveled a spoonful of eggs and two sausages after it, and headed into the lodge.

The program staff filled a long table near the fire and its tentative heat. Their bleary eyes and half-hearted yawns mimicked my own fatigue. The adventure of sleeping on a cot in a cabin had started to wear off. If given the chance, I'd sleep on a real mattress for two days without stopping.

Justin's gaze tracked me from the other side of the room where he sat nearest the fire, sipping a steaming mug of coffee. Mark had eaten early and left to deal with a possible bear sighting. JJ jerked his head in greeting when he spotted me. I smiled. My legs propelled me in that direction, but I slowed halfway there.

You never eat with us, Justin had said in the Jeep. On weekends, you hang out with your brothers.

JJ and Mark had become a kind of haven I'd been retreating to in the aftermath of losing my job, Nathan, and financial freedom. I swallowed. Perhaps it was time to fix my self-orientation.

With a quick turn to the right, I sat down next to Sione, the burly Tongan who oversaw the waterfront. Despite the nip of the chilly morning, he wore his usual pair of swimming trunks with a loose t-shirt and flip-flops. Next to him, Hollis, a blond, long-haired Californian, tossed pancakes into his mouth by the forkful. Troy sat across from me. At first he stared, and then he averted his eyes, swallowing heavily.

Once I settled in, I reached for a bottle of syrup and tried to ignore the now-quiet conversations. As nonchalantly as possible, I dashed syrup across my plate and set it back, as if I did this every day. Were they staring at me? I couldn't tell. Certainly felt like it.

"Hey, Megan," Emmett called from down the table. I perked up. "Are pancakes with syrup the latest breakfast fad?"

A few of them snickered. *Ah. So they want to test me.* After growing up with Mark and JJ, I knew enough about the male world to get by. *Oh, no. You won't get the best of me.* I rolled a sausage into a pancake, chomping a bite from it with a smirk.

"Nope. But freshly made pigs in blankets are back in, fellas."

"At least the pancakes were cooked all the way," said someone from the end. Another voice piped up after him.

"Not even burned!"

"My taste buds had seizures when they saw we weren't having cereal."

Although they nudged each other, laughing at their own jokes, I saw the careful attention in their expressions. Would I banter back? Or take it personally?

"Keep it up," I called back. "I can burn or undercook anything anytime I want!"

To my surprise, they laughed. The fervor died down until Sione elbowed me in the arm.

"So, Megan," he drawled, eyes flickering briefly to Troy. "I hear you're single."

A snigger came from down the table. Troy choked. My cheeks flared with sudden heat. A teasing, challenging note thickened in Sione's voice. Down the row, staff members turned away, lips pressed together to keep from laughing.

"Yes," I drawled, slicing into a pancake with the edge of my fork. "The last one told me to get into the kitchen and fix him a sandwich."

Sione tilted his head back and released a rolling belly laugh. Troy smiled. Hollis snorted. A few others down the table chortled, releasing their suppressed mirth. Across the way, I could feel Justin's eyes on my back.

Conversation continued down the table as if I weren't there, resuming its usual comfortable prattle. Apparently, I had passed. Troy's eyes darted to mine and then back to his plate.

"How's medical going, Troy?" I asked.

"Good." He nodded, his throat bobbing as he swallowed. "Thanks for, uh, your help yesterday. Someone had a laceration at the waterfront. I'm glad Gary's okay."

"No problem. Are you enjoying Adventura?"

"Yep."

"Where are you from?"

"Massachusetts." He stood up, gathering his plate and forks. "Thanks for breakfast, Megan. Tasted really good."

He dashed off. I watched him go, bemused. Maybe it hadn't been *everyone* that had been awkward at the beginning. Just Troy. Sione leaned over, his burly arm brushing mine.

"He's young. We're trying to teach him to be a man. Problem is, he has a mad crush on you, palangi."

My lips twitched. "Just like the rest of you?"

Sione roared with laughter again, slamming me on the back with a meaty fist. "I like her!"

From the corner of my eye, I saw JJ crack a grin. Justin stared at his plate, frowning, and didn't look my way again. I leaned back against my chair, relieved. Maybe I could worm my way into their hearts.

One meal at a time.

~

THE HOT DAYS of late June whipped by on dry winds and afternoon thunderstorms. We passed through the third week of camp with the crackle of oil on a hot grill.

After I finished prepping a sheet cake for poker night dessert on Saturday afternoon, I wandered outside to find JJ and Emmett. We had a date with the canoes and the lake for the rest of the day. The collective sound of shouts from the waterfront drew me in. My flip-flops echoed off the commissary walls as I passed it.

Most of the staff stood at the end of the pier, which had started to sink low in the water. Three of them sat on the outer edge, legs dangling in the lake, holding something white in their laps. Hollis, his long blond hair fanning out around his face in wild disarray, stood at the end of the dock, arms bent and fists clenched. Everyone chanted his name. He closed his eyes. With a mighty leap, he threw himself into the water.

Belly-flop style.

He landed with a resounding *smack* on the surface of the lake. A pathetic wave followed him, splashing the staff lining the dock.

"Holy balls!" he screamed when he surfaced. Sione fell back, laughing hysterically when Hollis emerged from the lake with red arms and shoulders. The three men sitting down leaned in, whispering.

Amongst the chaos, Atticus spotted me and trotted down the dock. He stuck his wet nose in my hand in greeting.

"Hey, boy," I murmured, running a hand over his silky fur. He led me to the group, black coat shining in the late afternoon sunshine. I sidled up next to Justin.

"What's going on?"

A ratty ball cap sat backward on top of his head above his gray-blue eyes. He motioned with a nod to the group.

"Belly flop contest. We're trying to find someone who can beat Sione. JJ and I think it's impossible."

I eyed the massive Tongan man. In chest width and shoulder span alone he had a major advantage. But that thick, strong belly would probably slap the very molecules of water apart.

Three white signs shot into the air. Hollis flipped the judges off, rubbing his sore arms. Justin laughed, wiping tears from his eyes. The amusement rolled out of his chest, deep and beautiful.

"The judges only scored Hollis a three, a negative four, and a one. That's terrible. With that slap, he earned at least a seven."

"What are their scores based on?"

"Nothing. They just like to see Hollis lose his temper."

Hollis's face had flared bright crimson while he argued. The three judges bent over, guffawing. Hollis shoved one of them into the water, and the other two fell apart, howling. Emmett stepped up to the edge next, staring at the murky water.

"No shirt!" JJ called. "You can't wear a shirt and win!"

While the rest of them heckled Emmett for leaving his shirt on, Justin leaned in toward me. A hint of vetiver filled my nose.

"There's a technique to belly flops," he said. "Watch."

Emmett tossed his body off the dock but bent at the waist just before he hit the water. A spray of water misted the air without a smack. Justin shook his head.

"No good."

The judges awarded Emmett negative one, zero, and negative twenty-four points.

"What will they win?" I asked.

Justin snorted. "Eternal respect. I mean ... look at Sione. He's pure Tongan brawn. In surface area alone he wins."

Jameson, a counselor, stepped up next. He turned the jump into a dive at the last minute and surfaced to hisses and boos. Sione strutted around the dock, smug. Most of them were jeopardizing their own attempts.

But perhaps if *I* could get it just right...

I slid out of my flip-flops and peeled my t-shirt off, revealing a dark olive tankini beneath. Justin glanced over, then quickly looked away.

"What are you doing?" he asked.

"I want to try."

His mouth dropped open. "You're kidding."

"Nope."

I left my shirt folded on top of my flip-flops and walked down the pier. Another splash preceded raucous laughter. Toby, a counselor, surfaced with a cough.

"Disqualified," said a judge. "No visible redness or audible smack."

The hilarity bubbled down as I closed in.

"She's gonna do it."

"No way!"

"Go Iron Chef!"

Their diffuse whispers at my back gave me courage. Mark stepped up behind me. "Blister," he sang, clutching my shoulders. "You wanna try?"

"Yep."

The whispers of the crowd increased.

"She's going up against Sione!"

"He'd eat her for breakfast!"

"No way she'll do it. Ten on Sione."

"I'll take that."

Sione regarded me through tapered eyes. His lips perked up in a half-smile. "You think you can beat me?" he asked, his voice rumbling. His muscular pecs danced as he folded his arms across his chest.

"Yep."

"Little girl," he drawled, a burr of an accent in his voice. "I was born on an island in Tonga. We live on the water. It obeys me."

I grinned. "We'll see about that."

"All right, gentleman," JJ called over the simmering conversation. "We have a new contestant!"

Rampant applause rang over the lake. I couldn't tell if they were rooting for me or saw me as the underdog.

"All right, little Miss Thang," Sione said, slapping his hands together. "Let's see you command that water like a palangi princess."

I stood at the edge of the pier, my toes curled over the edge. The warm, wet, splintered wood felt rough against my feet. Most of the guys had just fallen off, arms spread wide. But I'd try something different. I closed my eyes and prayed I wouldn't scream.

Silence descended on the crowd. The anticipation pulsed like a strobe light. I crouched low, drew in a breath, and sprang into the air like a released coil. Midflight, I straightened, pressed my stomach out, held my arms and legs high, and closed my eyes.

The moment I hit the water, a wave of pain raced from my stomach to my chest, arms, and the side of my face. I barely sank. Based on the slap burning through my skin, it had been a perfect drop.

The sounds of wild yelling and hysterics worked through the water in my ears. I bit back a moan as I surfaced, pushing hair out of my face. The staff stomped and clapped, screaming my name. My legs, stomach, left ear, and left cheek burned like a forest fire.

JJ reached down and pulled me out of the water. He shook his head. "Good grief, Meg. Nice work!"

"She's bright red!"

"Look at her arms."

"She fell like a bag of cement."

Sione blinked, hands on his hips, as he stared at the spot where I'd landed in the water. I felt like throwing up.

"Damn," he said, shaking his head. "The girl wins."

Elated—and a little nauseated—I held up a dripping fist.

"I am girl power!" I cried.

As one, all three judges held up 89.34, 10, and 1,000. The ballistic cheers turned into chanting. I forced a grin, waved, and bit back a surge of vomit. Mark elbowed through the crowd.

"You all right? You're bright red! I've never been so proud."

My skin tingled. I didn't dare look. Hands clapped my shoulders and pounded me on the back in congratulations as I worked through them, headed for my flip-flops.

And then somewhere to retch.

"Seriously, Meg," JJ said, following just behind. "You all right?"

"I just need to sit down."

"Let her through," Mark said, scattering the crowd. "She needs to get a drink of water or scotch or something."

Justin waited at the edge of the crowd with my shirt and flip-flops. When I approached, Atticus whimpered and licked my hand. I pulled my shirt on, grateful to cover up. Justin dropped my shoes in front of my feet. They slapped the deck, and I winced in sympathy.

"That was the loudest sound I've ever heard," Justin said.

Once I slid into the flip-flops, I straightened my wet, crooked shirt. My stomach rumbled. Justin put a hand on the back of my neck and spun me around to face the group of men chanting my name.

"Welcome to the club, Megan Bailey," he said. "I think you're in."

After waving, I doubled over and vomited all over Justin's shoes.

~

Breakfast Requests from Program Staff

- *BACON.*
- *Bacon*
- *Fruit with bacon.*
- *Donuts. No sprinkles.*
- *Ten cheese grilled cheese sandwich. With bacon.*
- *Bacon burritos*
- *WINGS with bacon*
- *Pie. Breakfast pie okay. Bacon expected. Fruit welcome.*
- *Bacon nachos*
- *French toast*
- *"Omelet the size of my face" <— Unsure who wrote this.*
- *^ With bacon*

13

CLOSURE

Rain pattered against the windowpanes of the lodge after dinner the next Tuesday evening, accompanied by an occasional roll of thunder. Puddles collected in low sections of the trails, resulting in a slippery cement floor when the staff trooped inside. Justin built a warm fire in the big hearth, and the sweet scent of pine seeped through the room. These calm evenings at Adventura made me want to stretch the summer into forever.

The epic belly-flop had turned the tide of staff adoration wildly in my favor. Throwing up on Justin had only cemented my place in their Hall of Fame. Luckily, Justin had been gracious and jumped in the lake to rinse his feet off while I burned with embarrassment.

After I'd finished wrapping leftover pizza—thin crust to avoid burning in the fickle oven and ManStyle with only meat and cheese and bacon—in tinfoil, the back door opened. Hollis walked inside, raindrops sparkling in his long, blond hair.

"Hey, girl power."

As recompense for taking his belly-flop champion status, Sione had bestowed on me the new nickname *girl power*. Everyone adopted it. I didn't mind. Their constant teasing and now frequent mini-pranks warmed the icy layers of my post-Nathan heart.

"Thanks for dinner," he continued. "I appreciate you adding mushrooms to one of them for me."

I smiled. "No problem."

He stood on top of an old towel in the doorway. His fingers fidgeted with the bottom of his shirt as he turned his body away from me, half-facing the fridge.

"Something on your mind?" I asked.

He rushed forward, as if he'd just been waiting for permission, and leaned across the island. "Can I ask you a favor?"

"Sure."

"I need help with ... with a girl."

"Okay."

His shoulders slumped. "Her name is Mandy, and she's wonderful. She lives in Jackson City. I just ... I'm not sure how to ... ask her out. I had a bad breakup a few months ago." He winced. "I'm still not sure what went wrong."

"Did you break it off?"

"No, she did."

"Have you spoken with her since?"

"No."

"So you don't know why it happened?"

He shrugged. "Just came out of the blue. I keep worrying that I did something horribly wrong."

"Did something bad happen right before?"

He paused and shook his head. "No. Maybe she just rejected me, right? Or maybe it had nothing to do with me." He threw his hands in the air. "I don't know! But if I messed up, I may do it again with the next girl I date."

"Maybe you need to find out what happened before you move on."

"Call my ex?" he asked. "But she's crazy."

"Maybe it'll give you closure?"

"Closure," he repeated, humming the word deep in his throat as if he'd never heard it before. "Hmm."

I warmed to the idea as it spun through my mind. "Find out why the relationship went wrong. Talk to your ex and see what she says. Maybe if you find out why, you won't be so gun-shy to start another relationship."

He straightened. "Yeah. That could work, I think."

I smiled. "Give it a shot. Couldn't hurt anything, right?" My expression fell. "She's not a *total* psycho, is she?"

"Not that I'm aware of. Hasn't been convicted of any murders ... yet." A wide grin split his face. He tapped once on the island with his knuckles. "Thanks, Megan. I'll try that out."

He left as quickly as he'd come. I stared at a shiny square of leftover tinfoil on the counter and listened to my own words.

Maybe it'll give you closure.

Nathan filled my head like a balloon as I mopped the floor. Adventura kept me so busy I didn't think about him much anymore. But he loitered in every now and then, like a full bag of garbage that needed taking out.

~

AN HOUR LATER, I stared out at the soggy trees, my nose stinging with the dry scent of bleach. Maybe Hollis wasn't the only one that needed closure. I deserved a chance to respond to how Nathan had broken up with me. A rush of adrenaline made my fingers tingle. It would feel wonderful to tell Nathan how I'd felt that night.

You dropped me like a hot potato, I'd say. I really liked you. I went into debt to impress you. I worked hard, and you just gave up. You valued your career over our relationship, and that really hurt.

I rinsed out a washcloth and hung it over the sink's edge. Tonight, justice would be served.

Tonight, I would get my own closure.

Ten minutes later, I sat on my cot in a pair of warm sweats, yellow knee socks, and a fleece jacket. Two bars of service showed up on my phone.

"Please hold out," I murmured, fingers crossed as I found his name in my contacts and hit *call*. I really didn't want to make this call in the lodge or main office. Atticus curled up on the cot next to me, his head spilling into my lap. The phone rang in my ear. A little tremor moved every bone in my hands as I waited for Nathan to pick up. I closed my eyes and exhaled a long, deep breath, moving into the safe mountainous place I went to during yoga.

You gave up. Why did you give up? I would have fought for you. For us. How dare you break up with me for your career? I rehearsed my speech over and over again. The words, running through my head like a ticker tape, fueled my courage.

Just focus, Megan. Tell him how you felt. Find your closure.

A harried voice answered moments later. A crackle of static filtered through the line, but it eventually evened out.

"Yeah?"

I paused. "Uh ... Nathan?"

"Who is this?"

Surely it hadn't been *that* long. "Nate, it's Megan."

A beat of hesitation lingered in the dead air. "Megan?"

"Yes. Your ex-girlfriend?"

"Yeah, I know. Hi."

"You sound stressed. Everything okay?"

He exhaled a short, fast staccato. I could picture him shoving his hands through his hair. I didn't need to see him to know that he had a wild, cagey expression on his face.

"New York is crazy, Meg. It's just ... crazy."

"Do you want me to call later?"

The sound of a door closing preceded his response. "No, this is fine. I can talk for two minutes. Oh, hold on." His voice muffled. He returned thirty seconds later. "Sorry. I'm prepping for a meeting."

"We can do this later. I—"

"There is no later, Meg. There is *no* later."

"Oh. Really?"

He sighed. "Yeah."

My rehearsed speech slipped away like tendrils of smoke. I cleared my throat. Of all the responses I'd planned for, this frenetic uncertainty hadn't been one of them. What did *crazy* mean, anyway? Nathan loved intense jobs.

"Are you enjoying your promotion?" I asked.

"It's nonstop. There've been five other people in this position in the last year. Five. I worked eighty hours last week. I only slept like four hours every night."

I snorted. "Hope you get paid overtime."

"I don't. At least, I don't think I do. I wouldn't even know. I haven't checked my own bank account in ... I don't know how long."

I leaned forward and pressed my cheek to the gentle, warm fur on the top of Atticus's head. He snuggled close. Outside, the warm fall of rain continued, pattering in a gentle dance on my rooftop. How wonderful the forest smelled during a rainstorm.

"I've been through two assistants already," he continued. "It's only been a month. I forgot to eat two meals the other day. I think I have a UTI because I don't have time to rehydrate. I can't remember the last time I cut my hair."

"Nathan, that's so..."

"Intense?"

"Unlike you."

"Right?"

"Do you like it?"

"What do you mean?"

"The job. Do you like it?"

"No." He paused. "At least, I don't think I do. I don't even know."

"But isn't it your dream? Living in New York City. Working your way into an executive position. Sounds ideal, right?"

The words seemed to hang in the air between us. "I don't know anymore. I really don't. It's all so different than I thought. I mean ... I just don't know." He sighed. "Listen, enough about me. Can I help you with something?"

My mouth opened, but no words came out. Instead of a thirst for retribution, I felt a surge of compassion. Like me, he'd given much of his life to his career, sacrificing time, money, health, and even relationships. And now he faced a future that he'd created—had once desired, even—but that didn't promise happiness.

"Megan? You there?"

"Right." I jerked back to attention. "Sorry. Uh, listen, I won't take up a lot of your time. I'm just calling because ... well, I wanted to check on you. Maybe get a little closure on our relationship."

"I was kind of an ass."

I paused, running the words through my head twice before fully comprehending what he'd said.

"Wait. What?"

"Yeah ... about that night. I'm sorry for the way that happened. You're wonderful. You really are. I was caught up in the excitement of the promotion and just acted."

"Oh." Tears pooled in my eyes. Could he ever know how wonderful it felt to hear that? No matter how much I blamed myself, it hadn't been just me.

"Uh, thanks."

"Although I still hold that we weren't easy. Breaking up really was for the best, now that I see my job." He sighed. "Things really didn't work out the way I wanted, did they?"

My thoughts wheeled backward. Nate wanted an easy relationship with an elusive *it* factor. But maybe he'd had one valid point—we *hadn't* been easy. The forced dinner conversations. Romantic galas where we spent almost no time together. He only did cardio, while I lifted weights. My mind strayed to Justin, then to JJ and Mark. *Easy,* Nathan had said.

It made a lot more sense now.

"You were right, actually," I said. "We weren't easy. That doesn't mean we couldn't have made it work, but ... I don't think we were meant to be together either."

His voice dropped. "Yeah. But the good times were good."

"Yeah."

"Are you kidding?" he yelled. "I had a phone call with LA five minutes ago! Meg, listen, I gotta go "

"Of course. Thanks, Nate. Really."

"Yeah. You too. Good luck with everything."

The line went dead. I chuckled, turned it off, and dropped it into my lap.

"Goodbye, Nathan," I whispered.

Atticus groaned when I disturbed his nap by tucking the phone under my leg. I ran a hand down his long, muscular side, marveling that my heart felt light and free. The manic intensity of my thoughts slowed. For the first time in weeks, I felt as if I could finally put Nathan behind me.

With my hands tucked underneath Atticus's silky coat, I dozed to the patter of raindrops.

14

COMPLETE CHAOS

Fourth of July Checklist

- *Check oven for firecrackers. (Mark's prank war begins at midnight)*
- *Sleep with eyes open*
- *Plan meal for the Great Big Massive Fourth of July Extravaganza.*
- *Food ideas:*
- *White Sheet Cake flags. (The ones on Pinterest.)*
- *Bowl of fresh fruit*
- *Watermelon slices*
- *Lemonade*
- ~~*Sandwiches?*~~
- *Veggie tray*
- ~~*BBQ Chicken*~~
- *Hot dogs*
- *Buy 200 hot dogs. And buns.*
- *Buy burn ointment.*

The Fourth of July dawned with a mosaic sunrise of lavender, electric pink, and smudged-butter yellow. I stared at the clouds, my head craned back, enjoying the majesty of the mountains under such a sky. A perfect day to celebrate freedom.

After serving a successful breakfast of biscuits and gravy—only slightly congealed—I grabbed my phone.

Buttercream or whipped topping? Which one is a better frosting? I typed in a text to Lexie. Then I paused, thumb hovering over the screen. With a quick tap, I deleted her name and substituted Mom's. Lexie and I hadn't spoken since her betrothal—mostly my fault. She'd sent messages that I hadn't responded to. My heart turned to flame every time I thought about giving her up to Bradley.

Silly Megan. Buttercream wins every time.

I yanked the fridge open while texting. *We're feeding 50 campers and 20 staff. Assume 3 hot dogs per male. 200 enough?*

Yep. Mark alone can polish off 5 with chili.

Fresh fruit? I asked.

Nice try. How about potato chips?

Already bought, I replied, feeling smug. *And a triple recipe of potato salad.*

You are a wise woman.

I'm still setting out fresh fruit.

I grinned and set the phone aside. "Gonna be ready, blister?" Mark asked, speeding through the kitchen, a ring of keys jangling on his hip. "It's going to be amazing. And complete chaos. Prep yourself."

I gave him a thumbs-up, but he'd already left. I stood at the top of the kitchen, surveying my kingdom in anticipation. Three sheet cakes to whip up, frost, decorate, and cut. Potatoes and eggs to boil, peel, and cut. Hot dogs to assemble into a cooler. Fruit to slice. Lemonade to perfect. And, above all, watermelon to chill and then chop. I tied my apron strings in a confident, certain knot.

"Happy Fourth of July," I said with a grin and grabbed a bag of flour. "Chef Megan is in the house."

THAT AFTERNOON, campers scampered through the open meadow like chipmunks on caffeine. They swooped around with sparklers, trying to stab each other. Behind them sprinted harried counselors, desperate to avoid burns or flesh wounds.

I tossed a stack of paper plates on the end of the main picnic table. Food filled every open spot. I gazed at one of three perfectly frosted sheet cakes. On top, strawberries and blueberries formed the stripes of the American flag. To my relief, each cake had emerged from the oven fully cooked without a brown spot in sight. Maybe the stove was patriotic. Or my experiment with turning the cakes every seven minutes had paid off.

Sione, Justin, and Hollis conspired near the picnic table, speaking in hushed tones and glancing furtively at Mark. They held red solo cups filled with a tart but sweet lemonade.

"Our best bet is to hide firecrackers outside the outhouse and light the fuse when Mark is inside. He did that to me last year," Justin said.

"What about putting poppers underneath the toilet seat so when he sits down they all pop?" Sione asked.

Justin shook his head. "Risky. Someone could go in before him. Also—do you want to be the one that lifts that toilet seat?"

Sione grimaced.

"There's always the classic of lighting a chain of firecrackers and throwing them into his cabin." Hollis laughed as if he'd told a joke. "Hurts every time."

"You'll have to do something more unique than that," I said, flicking a pine needle off the table. Sione hooked a beefy arm around my neck and reeled me in.

"What do you have in mind, girl power?"

"Something original. Something he's never seen before."

Justin's eyes narrowed. "That's impossible. Mark has always been the prank champion. He knows all of them."

"Something *without* fireworks," I said. "He's expecting them, so he'll be on guard."

"But it's the Fourth of July." Hollis motioned around with a sweep of his arm. "Of course we have to go with the theme."

I shook my head. "I'm telling you—he'll be expecting it."

"She has a point," Justin said. "We need to take him by surprise."

"We could tape all his stuff to the ceiling."

"Put a fog horn under his bed so it sounds when he lays down."

They tossed ideas back and forth while I studied Mark. He played hacky sack with a group of five campers. The Clipboard of Power swung in his arm. He never lost sight of it.

Or let go of it.

"Or," I drawled, "you could do something with the Clipboard of Power."

All three grinned.

Hollis lifted a hand for a high five, which I supplied. "That's it," he said. "That's the one. We're going to mess with the Clipboard of Powah."

The radio on Justin's hip crackled. JJ's voice echoed from Mark, Justin, and Sione's nearby radios.

"Hey, gladiator, is Megan nearby?" JJ asked.

Justin pulled the radio off his belt. "Yeah," he said. "What's up?"

"I need to talk to both of you."

JJ's carefully controlled tone caught my attention. Justin met my gaze. "Where?"

"Staff tents. Oh, bring your Jeep keys."

Justin fell into step with me.

"On our way."

"Do your thing, gladiator." Hollis gestured between him and Sione. "We got this."

"Something happened," I said, breaking into a jog. "Or he would have said why he wanted us over the radio."

"Any chance this is a prank?" he asked.

"Yep. But we have to be sure."

Ten heavy canvas tents raised on wooden platforms littered the forest south of my cabin. JJ didn't need to be more specific when he said *staff tents.* I heard muffled groans as we approached and followed the sounds.

"JJ?"

"Over here!"

Justin and I arrived on the scene to find Troy lying on his back, his mangled right arm resting on his stomach. A broken bone in his wrist protruded against his skin, turning it white. Sweat beaded on his forehead. He clenched his teeth together with a moan of pain.

"Not a joke," Justin muttered.

"Nice work, Troy." I dropped to my knees at his side. "What happened?"

JJ bit his bottom lip. "We were, uh, debating who could climb higher up the tree. Technically, Troy won." His gaze darted to the fractured bone. "And lost."

"We need to splint it and get him to the ER. JJ, leave me your radio. Go to the medical cabin and find something to splint it with. Justin, discreetly tell Mark what happened and then bring your Jeep as close as you can."

Like insects in the light, they scattered. While I attempted to make Troy comfortable and performed a quick assessment of the injury, the sounds of the celebration rang in the background. A minute later, Mark jogged up.

"Justin just told me. Oh, man," he said, grimacing. "Troy, that looks terrible. Kind of awesome, but really terrible."

Troy swallowed, his breathing strained. "Thanks," he muttered, screwing his eyes shut.

JJ returned. He and Mark supported Troy while I splinted the broken arm to his chest. He paled while I secured it with a gentle knot. Seconds later, Justin pulled up on the other side of the trees, his tires crunching on the gravel.

"All right, Troy," I said, standing. "Let's get you to the ER."

After making Troy as comfortable as possible, I reached to pull the Jeep door closed. Mark grabbed my arm. I met his intent hazel eyes.

"Hurry back, little blister," he said. "You're Adventura's new medical officer now."

15

A LITTLE BREATHER

I stood at the window of the hospital waiting room a couple of hours later. In the background, a listless TV droned a news report. The quiet bustle of the hospital provided a soothing medical landscape. I sank into the familiarity again with relief.

"Thought I'd find you here."

A light tap on the door startled me. Mom filled the doorway wearing scrub pants and a plain t-shirt. Her badge hung from a lanyard around her neck.

"Hey," I said, turning around. "What are you doing here?"

"Just stopping by really quick to say *hi*. Mark texted me. I'm filling in at the ICU tonight. Where's Troy?"

"Went to surgery twenty minutes ago. Justin left to grab us some food. Are you all right?" I peered closer. What I originally thought was a ponytail was actually a short bob, cropped close to her head. Feather-like brunette strands lay in wisps around her face. "Did you ... did you cut off your hair?"

A wan smile crossed her lips.

"I did. You know what they say about a haircut making everything better? Well, that's kind of a lie. But I thought I'd try it out."

I blinked, unable to remember the last time I'd seen Mom without her usual locks. I couldn't recall a single instance.

"Wow."

She ran her fingers through it. "Do you like it?"

"I just ... I mean, yes. It's beautiful."

"You seem shocked."

"I am. I've never seen your hair shorter than your shoulders."

She folded herself into a nearby chair. "I thought it was time for a change."

"Do you like it?"

She shrugged. "Cuts down prep time by thirty minutes. But then, I have to wash it every day. Not that it's difficult or anything, but it's one more thing to do."

She didn't answer my question.

"How is work?" I asked.

"Slow tonight. But that's a good thing."

A span of silence hummed between us while I debated whether or not I should ask about her and Dad. She decided before I could ask.

"So ... I wasn't sure if I should tell you, but ... your father and I are taking a little breather," she said. A hint of tears misted her eyes, thickening her voice. My breath caught.

"When?"

"Started last week."

Why didn't you tell us? I wanted to ask but swallowed it back. "What does *a little breather* mean?" I asked instead.

She held up a hand. "Nothing final or anything. We just decided to try officially living apart even though we're not around each other much anymore. Our therapist suggested it. I've been hesitating, but we've tried everything else."

"Is it ... is it helping?"

Desperation tainted my voice. Mom squeezed my hand.

"I don't know. The therapist assures us that these things take time..." She pressed a hand to her heart. "I don't know."

To my surprise—and relief—she didn't weep or wilt into a pile of regret. She sat there, staring at the floor. A flicker of hope rose from the depths of my fear. The *D* word hadn't quite entered the picture yet. There was still hope. As much as I hated it, I clung to it, that traitorous, slippery emotion.

"Do you have a place to stay?" I asked.

"I'm at the house. He's ... somewhere in the old trailer."

Dad's clunky, rusted trailer was his pride and joy. It smelled like fish and creaked with every small gust of wind, but he adored it.

Another silence filled the space between us. This time I let it ride, too focused on my own questions to care. In the end, what could I say? Justin had been right; this wasn't my fight. As much as I wanted it to be.

"Keep me updated, will you?" I finally asked.

"Of course."

"Okay, so, I went to Subway because—"

Justin stopped mid-stride, holding a plastic bag and a drink container. His gaze fell first on my mother, half-hiccupping from forcing her tears back, and then on me. No doubt I looked confused. Or frightened. Or some odd conglomeration of both. His eyes widened. He stepped back.

"Uh, sorry. I didn't—"

Mom stood up. "Hello there, Justin!" she said, wiping the last vestiges of tears from her cheeks with a smile. "It's always wonderful to see you. Are you still keeping track of my troublesome boys? They're a handful. Don't I know it!"

"Of course, Mrs. Bailey. Your haircut looks great."

She touched the nape of her neck. "Oh. Thank you. It's a bit shorter than I like. I hate it, actually."

He held up a Subway bag. "Fortunately for you, I brought the fix-all to your problems."

"Oh? What's that?"

He rifled through the bag and pulled out a second paper bag. "Cookies. But not *just* cookies. Chocolate chip. They fix everything."

Mom laughed, restoring a sense of youth to her countenance. "Thank you," she said, accepting one. "I think you must be right."

He motioned to me with a jerk of his head. "Thank Megan. You're eating one of hers."

"Well, I better head out," Mom said. "Thanks so much, Meg, for listening. And Justin, the biggest thanks goes to you for fixing all my problems with this fantastic cookie."

"Anytime, Mrs. Bailey."

Mom reached down and squeezed my shoulder. "Love you."

Justin and I stared at each other until the sound of my mother's shoes faded away. He pulled in a deep breath, sat in the chair next to mine, and tossed the remaining cookies onto my lap.

"Start with a cookie," he said. "You look like you could use it."

~

THAT EVENING, Mark and I stood just inside the tiny medical cabin, tucked away in the trees behind the lodge. Late shadows moved across the floor. A cot, a desk for charting, and a random assortment of cupboards filled the cabin. The smell of hand sanitizer permeated the room.

"So ... being the medical officer is pretty straightforward," he said, glancing around. "You've handled the most complicated patients already. The daily splinters and bloody knees shouldn't be too difficult."

I pulled open a few drawers, rifling through the contents. Mark swung a loop of keys around his index finger. After I finished perusing the cupboards, I nodded.

"Should be easy enough," I said.

Mark gave me a half-smile. "Look, I know I'm asking a lot. Running the kitchen *and* medical will be tricky sometimes, but most of the issues here are minor. We have to have a licensed person on staff, and you have a crap ton of certifications, right?"

If he only knew.

"Yeah. I do."

"Great. I've talked to the program staff, and they've promised to help out at mealtimes if needed."

I held out a hand. "I get a radio, right?"

He handed me Troy's old radio with a grin. "Obviously. Just, uh, keep it with you all the time. Like sleep, bathroom, exercise, kitchen. Oh, and no more weekday trips to Pineville."

I lifted an eyebrow. "I'm on camp arrest?"

"Yes."

"Lovely."

"You gotta stay here when campers are present. I will not lose this place because of litigation. I've basically sacrificed myself to it like the Old Testament."

"Are you going to stop calling me little blister now?"

He snorted. "Fat chance. You *are* the blister. Listen, I gotta go do a quick camp inspection, make sure no one smuggled firecrackers in. By the way, have you seen my clipboard?"

After the long day—and the exhausting conversation with Mom—I didn't think I had any energy left to smile, but a glimmer of amusement took me by surprise. *Way to go, Hollis and Sione.*

"Nope."

He muttered a swear word under his breath as he turned to leave, eyes darting all over the cabin. "Could have sworn—"

"Hey, Mark?"

He stopped and turned around. In the dim light, he looked just like Dad.

"Yeah?"

"Do you know what's going on with Mom and Dad right now?"

The playful expression on his face faded. His pond-water eyes seemed to collect the shadows in the room. For a brief moment, I thought I saw in him the same ache I felt.

"What do you mean?"

Our eyes locked, as if we could ascertain how much the other one knew by visual assessment. Mark was the older of the twins and bore the responsibility of the eldest sibling in every regard.

"You know, don't you?" I asked.

He started to leave again. "Don't be crazy, Meg. They're fine."

"They're *not* fine."

He stopped halfway out the door, shoulders tight.

"Whatever is happening between them has nothing to do with us, okay?" he said. "Just let them figure it out."

I started forward. "Mark, it's getting worse. They're living apart now. It doesn't make sense." I pressed a hand to my forehead. "How can they just fall out of love? Can you at least tell me what you know?"

He shook his head with an exasperated sigh. A tight edge cut through his voice. "Let it go, Meg."

"Mark!"

"What?"

"Talk to me about this. Please? Mom asked me not to talk to anyone about it. But I can't hold it in anymore. I'm not sure how much JJ knows, but I *know* you must know something already. Please?"

He hesitated, pinning me with his stare. "Fine. What do you want to know?"

I folded my arms across my middle, fending off a sudden chill. Outside, darkness had started to fall in earnest, coating the world in deepening shadows. I thought I wanted answers, but now that he'd offered them, I couldn't shake the feeling I was plunging deeper into the rabbit hole.

"When did you find out they were having problems?" I asked.

He swallowed. "A year ago Dad and I went fishing. He seemed quieter than usual and really distracted."

I scoffed. He must have been almost comatose. Dad didn't speak much even when he had something to say.

"He told you then?" I asked.

"I asked him about it. I'd noticed that things seemed weird. They didn't talk much. Mom kept texting me to ask the most random questions. That kind of stuff."

"What did he say?"

"That things had been strained between them after Mom started the flight-nurse job at St. John's. But he said they'd work through it." He threw his hands in the air. "And here we are."

"Was it this bad then?"

He shrugged. "Not sure. I was caught in the middle of it for a while, but that only made things worse, so I've left it alone. It's not our business."

"Why didn't anybody tell me?"

"It's not exactly something to talk about over the phone. I figured the day would come when they'd decide and everyone would know then. Why burden you with it sooner? There was a chance they'd figure it out."

My heart squeezed as if he'd just wrapped it in barbed wire and it still had to beat. He put a hand on my shoulder, shaking me lightly.

"I'm sorry, Meg. Nothing can save them but them. Trust me. I've tried."

Tears filled my eyes. I felt filleted open, as vulnerable as an injured two-year-old seeking reassurances. Justin had said the same thing, but it didn't feel any better coming from Mark.

"But what if they decide it's not worth saving? What about *us*?"

He reached out and pulled me into a warm hug, just like when I was a little girl. Tears dribbled down my cheeks.

"Then that's what they decide," he whispered. "And we'll always have each other. We'll have them, too. Just not in the same way."

"That's not fair."

"I know."

I squeezed him as hard as I could. When I pulled away, he ruffled my hair. "Keep your chin up. JJ and I won't go anywhere, all right?"

I nodded.

"You're a good blister," he said with a brief, jaunty grin. "A pain, but a good pain."

I laughed. "Thanks, Mark."

With a wink, he ducked away, fading into the emerald foliage with little more than the whisper of his feet on the trail. I didn't feel better. The deepening fear in my chest seemed to swallow the last of my hope. Although Mark hadn't said it, I'd seen it in his eyes.

He didn't believe they'd work it out.

16

DESPERATE MEASURES

As it turned out, being the camp nurse and the staff chef wasn't as bad as I'd expected.

It was far worse.

Campers injured themselves at the most inopportune times. Anything from open blisters to splinters to swollen bug bites. I'd slap antibiotic ointment and band-aids on kids while praying my cornbread and chili didn't burn. Once they left, I'd sprint to the lodge to keep up with meal prep.

The last half of the summer closed in. On Monday morning of the sixth week of camp, the smallest group arrived—only twenty boys. Four of the ten counselors left to vacation for the week, not needed with so few participants. While stirring a pot of meat sauce, I grabbed my ringing phone and answered an unknown number.

"Hello?"

"Is this Megan Bailey?"

Something about the tinny, distant quality of the voice set my hair on edge. I hesitated.

"Uh, yes."

"Wonderful. My name is Jameson. I work with Traveler's Credit Card."

My stomach melted. "Oh." I cleared my throat. "Hi."

"We're calling in regards to your missed payment for the month of July.

According to our records, this is the second payment you've missed. Your minimum payment due has now risen to—"

"I lost my job!" I cried, then bit down on my knuckle. "Sorry. Didn't mean to scream at you. Look, I know that I haven't paid the minimum due, but the truth is that ... I can't."

Jameson paused. "You can't?"

I grimaced. Why had I said that? Surely he didn't want to hear the truth if that's what it came to. "I was laid off at work, and now I'm seeking ... new employment."

"When were you laid off?"

I swallowed. "At the end of May."

"And have you filed for unemployment?"

"No."

"Are you actively looking for new job opportunities?"

"Of course."

"I'm sorry for your loss," he said, sounding annoyed, "but that doesn't change your minimum balance. You've missed two consecutive payments. And now that I know you don't have work, I've frozen the account to keep you from using it again."

I ran a trembling hand through my hair.

"Listen, what if I promise you that I can make a payment next month?" I asked. "When is it due?"

"August tenth."

My flight back home left August first, which wouldn't leave enough time to start a job and be paid by the tenth. I growled under my breath. Since Jodie hadn't found any hiring bonuses, the only way I could promise to make any kind of payment was to borrow money—not likely given the family's current circumstances—or leave Adventura early.

Both options left a metallic taste in my mouth.

"Are you there, Miss Bailey?"

"Yes. Sorry. What happens if I don't pay the minimum payment due by August tenth?"

"Your bank will be notified, and we'll give you to a debt collector. Trust me. They never stop calling."

"Fine," I snapped. "I'll pay ... something by then."

"You will?"

"Yes."

"Even though you just informed me that you don't have a job?"

"I will by then. I'm working with a recruiter."

"Do you have any money to put down as a show of good faith?"

"I wish. Well ... I have twenty bucks but—"

"Great. I'll make a note of this conversation and plan on seeing that good faith payment come through within the next couple of days. I will speak with you again on August tenth, Miss Bailey. Thank you for your time."

The line went dead. I dropped the phone to my side, allowing my mind to speed away. Did I dare tell Mom or Dad? No. Out of the question right now. Mark and JJ had no money. None of the Health and Happiness Society had over five hundred dollars lying around that I knew of—I hadn't exactly kept in touch with them. Could I lose my house? My car? My credit? I didn't want to find out. I only had one option.

With heavy fingers, I clicked through my phone. It only rang twice.

"This is Jodie Renner with EveryHealth."

"Jodie, it's Megan."

"Oh. Hello again. I didn't expect to hear from you this soon."

"Uh ... there's been a slight change of plans."

"Yes?"

I closed my eyes. "Find me a job. *Any* job."

She paused. "Okay," she drawled. "Starting when?"

My tongue stuck to the top of my roof like sandpaper. "Uh ... anytime."

"I'll be in meetings for the rest of the day, but I'll compile a list when I'm back. Expect to hear from me Monday afternoon, all right?"

Fabulous. A whole weekend to dwell on this conundrum. I swallowed.

"Yeah, sounds great. Thanks, Jodie. I really appreciate the help."

"No problem. Talk to you soon."

The sound of the dial tone filled my ear, sounding an awful lot like the dead hum in my chest.

What was I going to tell Mark and JJ?

The debt pressed into my chest like a heart attack for the rest of the day. Every moment I wasn't searching for another option—Could I sell my car long-distance? Did I own any jewelry I could pawn?—I spent the rest of it swearing I would never again let my finances fall on the back burner.

Or plummet because of a guy.

"Hey, Emmett. Will you grab that pot of pasta and take it off the burner?" I called later that evening, just five minutes before dinner. "This meat sauce will burn if I leave it."

Emmett leaped up from where he sat on a bench in the dining area and hurried into the kitchen. "Sure thing, girl power."

"Sorry. I was called into medical to fix a laceration."

"No problem."

Staff members streamed into the dining hall from all parts of Adventura, sweaty, hot, sunburned, and starving. A couple of them filled their water bottles at the sink while telling me stories about annoying campers.

"The kid cried because his feet got wet. I don't understand. It's a lake. With *water*," Sione muttered.

"Maybe he didn't want to ruin his shoes?"

Sione snorted. "He was barefoot."

He tossed a water bottle in the recycling can before banging his way into the dining room. Several other staff members came in, talking to me over each other.

"...then the little kid punched the big kid. It was pretty sweet. Don't look at me like that, Megan. I stopped it ... eventually. He deserved it. It was a true David-and-Goliath story..."

"So there I was, on top of the climbing tower..."

Spaghetti sauce and onions bubbled on the stovetop while I listened, commenting here and there while the kitchen filled with the scent of oregano and tomatoes. I toggled three different conversations and two side dishes at the same time. The distraction from my debt was a welcome relief.

"Hey, JJ," I called into the dining room. "Start setting out plates of butter, will you? Thanks!"

He leaped to his feet, abandoning an ongoing game of poker that had been running at mealtimes for at least a week.

JJ and Emmett bustled around the kitchen under my orders as I orchestrated the symphony of dinner. Their willing hands cut down my work by half. I was just tasting the spaghetti sauce after adding a dash of brown sugar when Mark burst into the kitchen. Justin followed close behind, grease on his hands from working on the camp truck. He headed for the sink. I rolled up the window into the lodge as the staff gathered.

"Dig in, gentlemen," I called, ringing the bell with a satisfying *whack*.

The staff flooded forward, scrambling for plates, forks, and fresh rolls. Behind me, something slapped the island. I spun around to see a folded map next to the second bowl of noodles.

"Found this over the weekend," Justin said. "Thought you might be interested."

"A map?"

I wiped my hands on my apron before picking it up. When the creased, rain-resistant material unfurled, an aerial view of the mountains surrounding Adventura lay before me. Justin reached over my shoulder and pointed out camp. A delicious hint of vetiver mingled with the heady tinge of automotive oil.

"Here we are," he said.

He pointed to where the river flowed out of the canyon. A blue dot indicated the lake. His fingertip slid up the canyon and over to the right. A network of trails rambled like spider legs along the mountain ridge.

"Check this out—two trails lead up Custer Mountain," he said. "I thought there was only one."

I tapped on the left trail. "This western trail looks faster."

"No way. Check out that elevation profile. Eastern would be faster."

"Too many switchbacks. It's at least two miles longer."

A hint of challenge tightened his tone. "I disagree."

My own pride rose to the occasion. The only way to know who was right would be to test it. How delicious it sounded—conquering something tangible while the rest of my life fluttered to ash in the background.

"Wanna bet on it?" I asked, drawing out the budding idea. Justin canted his head to the side.

"Bet?"

"Yeah. Let's make a bet. I'll take the short route. You take the long. We'll leave at the same time. Whoever gets to the top first wins."

Justin's eyes gleamed.

"You got it, girl power. What's the prize?"

Since I officially had zero dollars to my name—having already promised the twenty dollars to Traveler's Credit Card—I cast about for something of high value. My eyes landed on the smorgasbord of food the staff had piled onto plates with reckless abandon.

"If I win, you cook dinners for the next week," I said.

He ran his tongue over his teeth. "That's it?"

"That's a lot!"

"Let's make it more interesting."

A thrill shot down my spine. The staff stared at us from the window, silent, hands poised halfway to their plates.

"How?"

"Fifty bucks *and* I make dinner for a week."

I swallowed. He had no idea how much fifty dollars was asking.

"If you win?" I asked.

"Fifty bucks and you ... clean all the biffies."

A couple of men behind us sniggered. The biffies—or outdoor toilets—were cramped wooden shacks with a toilet on top of a hole in the ground. Still, they had to be wiped down with bleach and restocked every week. Not only did they reek, but flies swarmed them. Would it be worth it?

Definitely.

With a flash of inspiration, I recalled my talk with JJ on top of the cliff. *His family is loaded. Lives in this big mansion in California. He's old money, I guess.* Desperate times called for desperate measures, didn't they?

"No," I said.

His eyebrows shot halfway to his hairline. "No?"

"Five *hundred* dollars."

A collective *ooh* came from the staff, preceding the chorus of dissents that rang in my head.

"Girl has balls," someone sang.

"She's insane."

"No one can beat Justin on a mountain."

"She's betting five hundred dollars with the gladiator?"

Their murmurs did little to dissuade me. My heart pattered like a bird in flight. If I won—which I would—his money would solve everything. I could meet the minimum balance on my debt by August tenth without leaving Adventura early. Jodie could get me into the right job instead of a last-minute desperate job.

Justin studied me before sticking out his hand.

"Agreed."

I accepted, ignoring the smirk that sent his dimple into a deep groove.

"You're on, girl power. You and me. Saturday morning."

I grinned. Me on the mountain? I'd been trail running with JJ almost every morning. Climbing and swimming every Saturday. Hiking with the twins every Sunday. I had this—and my debt issues—in the bag.

~

SATURDAY DAWNED with a big sky evenly funneled into a sliver by the mountains. Not a single cloud loitered in sight. The crisp, heady scent of pine needles drifted into my little cabin, calling to me. Eager to get on the trail, I shucked the sleeping bag off and scrambled for my hiking boots.

"Hey," JJ said when I hustled out of my cabin ten minutes later, finishing off an energy bar. He jogged to my side, his hair unbound and wet on his shoulders.

"Hey." I swallowed the last bite. "I was just on my way to the kitchen to grab my lunch."

JJ nodded toward the stream. "Justin's at the trailhead now. So is the rest of the staff. Oh, and I brought you these."

He extended four black packets to me. A bright crimson font across the front said, *The Gel Guru presents Black Cherry.*

"What are they?" I asked, glancing at the back. No list of ingredients. Minimal packaging with frayed edges and skewed font. "Are these black market or something?"

"Energy gels. A running buddy of mine is trying to get into it. He's testing this recipe, so he's not sure how well it works. Said something about extract of ginseng and a new caffeine mixture."

"Sounds ... intense."

"Want to try it out? You could give him some feedback. He wants to go wide with it but needs to know if it requires more ingredients, or fewer. And..." He paused. "Well ... let's just say you might need the extra boost."

My right eyebrow rose. "What's that supposed to mean?"

"Justin is the best hiker we have here."

"Better than you?"

"I'm a climber, not a hiker. There's a big difference. But yes, even better than me. Mark, too."

A shot of anxiety raced through me. Maybe I'd made this hasty bet without all the facts. Anyone that could beat JJ could beat me.

"He's a lowlander," I said, brushing it off. "I'll be fine. I grew up in the mountains."

"Not a lowlander anymore. He's been living in Jackson City for the past year. Look, I've hiked with him before. He has lungs the size of hot-air balloons. He'll dominate those extra two miles. Probably run up the whole thing and then back down even faster."

A shout from the stream caught our attention. Mark stood in the trees, waving for us. "We're waiting!" he called.

"Coming!" I said, shoving the gels in my bag as JJ and I started walking. JJ put a hand on my back.

"Just ... don't set your heart on this, okay?"

"It's $500. My heart is absolutely set on it."

And so is my future, I thought, setting my jaw.

"And the biffies," he quipped. "Don't forget how fun it will be to clean those."

"I'll win. I have to."

He said no more as we strode through the trees, but his silence told me everything.

"You ready for this, girl power?" Justin asked as we approached. He wore a pair of gray shorts and a loose t-shirt. The muscles in his legs seemed even more pronounced. I recalled his morning swim at the lake with a little blush and dismissed JJ's warnings.

"I was born ready," I said, cracking my neck.

Five hundred dollars, I told myself. Just get through the pain to get the gain.

Everyone gathered at a split in the trail a few yards from the stream, which we'd just crossed. Although they kept their voices low, I could hear them placing bets. Only a few went in my favor. Sione waved a stack of fives at me, no doubt to indicate his loyalty. Mercenary motivations aside, I wanted to make these guys proud of me again.

At any rate, it couldn't hurt *more* than the belly-flop.

Atticus stood between us, tail swinging, mouth open in a perpetual pant. "You take the dog," Justin said, nudging Atticus closer. I sank my fingers into his silky fur and didn't disagree. Adventura was private land, so the trail had been mostly unused. A neglected trail posed many dangers. Having Atticus with me would ease some of my worries.

"Thanks."

"May the best hiker win," Justin said. I tried not to focus on the rough feel of his callused hands against mine as we shook.

"I will."

He laughed, heading off onto his trail. Atticus watched him go, then looked up at me.

"C'mon, boy." I ruffled his fur. "Let's go."

The staff cheered as I spun around and headed for my own trail.

"Get him, girl power!"

"Beat the gladiator."

"Make us proud!"

Their calls faded into the background as I strode down the trail. If I could win a belly-flop competition, I could win this bet. I *would* win this bet and the freedom that making a big payment would bring.

Or so I hoped.

~

A NAGGING TUG made itself known in my stomach as I began the ascent up the steep mountainside, sliding on the occasional waterfall of loose rock. What if I failed to make it to the top? What if I was in over my head like JJ had suggested?

"No," I said, shaking my head. I wouldn't even *think* it. Karen's face when she let me go swam through my mind.

Then again, sometimes things didn't go the way I planned.

Imagining Justin powering his way up the other trail served as steady motivation for the first twenty minutes. One fiber at a time, the muscles in my legs warmed up. The trail climbed a steep pitch from the start. Within the first half hour, I felt like I'd climbed thirty flights of stairs. My lungs begged for air. Atticus stood on top of a boulder, peering at me as if to say, *Come on, silly human. We've just begun.*

"I'm ... coming..." I panted.

When I stopped at the rock, I propped my hands on my waist. I couldn't do this for seven miles and maintain a competitive pace. Although I was loath to admit it, JJ's energy gels called to me. I preferred hiking mountains on my own energy.

But maybe today's extenuating circumstances merited a little ... boost.

Reaching into a pocket, I grabbed a pouch, tore it open with my teeth, and downed it in one gulp. The saccharine taste of cherries and something metallic filled my mouth. I swallowed, chugging half a bottle of water with it. The aftertaste coated my tongue with a dry, chalky taste.

"Yuck." I wiped my mouth off with my sleeve. "These better be worth it."

A sharp snap broke the air when I started again. I paused, breath held. When I moved my eyes down, not daring to breathe, I confirmed my suspicion.

"A broken shoelace? Seriously?"

Two frayed ends of my shoelace hung over opposite sides of my right shoe, having broken apart right in the middle. Atticus trotted up to my side, sniffing into my shoe as I pulled it off. He recoiled. I rolled my eyes.

"That's your own fault," I muttered, my pack sliding off my shoulders. I sat on the trail and reached down, yanking the laces free with sharp, jerky movements. After two attempts, I tied a firm knot in the broken strings and re-laced the threads. They fell short, leaving two holes unfilled. The back of my foot slipped out of the shoe every now and then. *That'll be annoying after a few miles,* I thought.

"C'mon, Atty. Let's go."

I started up the trail but stopped ten feet later. The sound of four pattering paws didn't race to pass me. I turned around to find an empty trail. The leaves on the quaking aspens fluttered like thin coins in the breeze.

"Atty?"

I returned to the same spot and peered into the bushes. No sign. Not a single stirring of life.

"Not funny, Atticus. Come!"

A bluebird fluttered by, chased by another. They swooped past me, disappearing into the foliage.

"Atticus?"

I tromped into the bushes, shoving scrub oak aside, wresting brambles and knee-high wildflowers. When I stopped to unwind a strand of hair from a high branch, I froze. In the distance to my right came a faint bark.

"Atticus," I yelled, turning. "Atticus, come!"

The bark sounded again. I yanked my hair free and charged through the weeds. Ten minutes later, I stumbled on an old tree hiding in a copse of aspens. Atticus pranced along the base of it, barking with fits of aggression. In the lowest branches chattered a squirrel, its puffy tail flicking behind it like a horse.

"Seriously?" I grabbed his collar. "Let's go."

He wheeled around at my insistence, trotting through the high grass with an occasional glance back. The wild, untamed beauty of the meadows sprawled in disorienting skirts of variegated viridian and mossy green. The clump of trees on the left looked exactly like another clump of trees to the right. Various animal footpaths meandered through the space. I'd been so intent on not losing Atticus that I hadn't searched for landmarks. Disoriented by the *sameness* of it all, I stopped.

Atticus vaulted a high clump of wildflowers and headed north. I threw my hands in the air and followed. With any luck, he'd know where to go.

After another fifteen minutes of careful searching—and four attempted butterfly snacks—Atticus found the trail. We started our ascent a second time. Within minutes of reclaiming our path, a heady buzz sprinted through my legs. I pushed hard and fast, feeling the energy course through me like neon lights. Perhaps JJ's friend really had something with these gels. I'd have to tell him to keep the recipe.

We settled into a steady hour of uninterrupted hiking. The sharp mountain walls and heavy pitch of the trail required all my effort. Thanks to low traffic, Atticus and I lost the trail several times and had to backtrack, wasting precious time. In my bragging, I hadn't paid as much attention to the grade as I should have, but with the help of the gels, I pressed hard.

On the first outcropping, I stepped off the trail and peered down the mountainside. The height of our climb gave me vertigo. The edge dropped into a sheer rock face that plunged into the river. The canyon unfurled, carved by the distant whitecaps of the frothy water and the bushy peaks of the evergreens.

"Three miles," I murmured to Atticus, who peered down the side. I playfully swatted his face. "We finally made good time once you stopped chasing squirrels."

I grinned, grabbed a second energy gel, and slurped it down. A slow start notwithstanding, Atty and I had this hike in the bag.

~

AN HOUR, two miles, and three lost trail moments later, I lurched to a stop.

The top of Custer Mountain loomed high in the distance, a pillar of granite and stone. Half a mile ahead, the timberline disappeared into a field of slate and shale that led to the final ascent. The intense sunlight bounced off the pale rock faces.

Sweat coated my shirt and back, dripping down my arms in hot trails. The sun beat relentlessly hard this high. Every breath seemed to give me less oxygen. I glanced at my watch. Five miles completed. Only two left. My stomach churned, so I grabbed my bottle and swigged. Water leaked from the corners of my mouth and dribbled down my jaw. My unusually insatiable thirst left me only one more bottle. I'd never felt thirst so strong. Water had never tasted so refreshing.

After pouring the rest of the water into the bowl I carried for Atticus, I spun the lid back on and straightened up, surveying the soft meadows. The grasses waved in the gentle breeze, scattered with nodding wildflowers. Atticus finished drinking and pounced on a wandering moth, his jaws snapping. I put a hand to my still-rumbling stomach and peered up at the azure, cloudless sky. One day I'd come back up here and take time to enjoy the bigness of it all. A yawn tickled my jaw. I reached back for another energy gel, but my hand came back empty. Had I already eaten all three?

"C'mon, Atty," I said, replacing the pack. "Let's beat your human. I have a credit card to pay off and brothers to keep happy."

Just as I headed back to the trail, an irritated cramping in my bowels caught me by surprise. I paused. It soon passed, and I started hiking. Within minutes, my belly spasmed again. I had time to scramble into the trees before I lost all control. Ten minutes later, I returned, my stomach still in prickly stitches.

"Awesome," I muttered to Atticus. "Nothing helps a hike like grumpy bowels."

Atticus waited for me, ears perked, on the trail. When I stepped up to his side, he trotted away, tail swinging. But now, with my abdomen on the warpath, every step uphill felt like a small mountain. Despite my previous determination, my energy flagged. I trudged forward, my toes dragging in the dirt. Half an hour passed, and I'd only gone half a mile. Twenty yards away, the shale field began. The grass clumps had thinned out. A hawk soared overhead.

"Lunch," I murmured, with an edgy sense of panic. I needed to eat but had no time. The last thirty minutes should have gotten me at least a mile, if not more.

Still plodding, I reached into my backpack and groped for the two PB&J's I'd packed, but my fingers only brushed canvas at the bottom. I paused, then yanked the backpack strap off my shoulder and pulled it forward.

"No," I said, peering into the almost-empty pack. "No. Way."

I closed my eyes. I'd completely forgotten to grab lunch! JJ had side-railed me with his energy gels, and then Mark had called for us. All I had was a couple water bottles for Atticus, an old stick of jerky, an applesauce packet, and—eureka! Another energy gel. My stomach gurgled again. I snatched a small package of biodegradable toilet paper and dashed into the trees just in time. When I returned, Atticus nudged my pack with his nose.

"Yeah, I know," I said, ripping the top of the energy gel off with my teeth. "I'm hungry, too."

With the gel halfway to my mouth, I paused. JJ's words floated back through my mind. *He's testing this current recipe, so he's not sure how well it works.* Energy gels were packed with electrolytes and sugar and sometimes caffeine. They often caused gastrointestinal distress. This untested recipe could be worse than usual.

Especially during intense workouts.

I recalled the syrupy taste as I'd forced the others down. My gut seemed to roll over again. A dry, dense field of sand trickled down my throat. No wonder I'd been so thirsty! Energy gels required water to break down.

I tossed the gel back into my pack with a growl.

"Great. I did this to myself."

Going further now would be risky for several reasons—there was no cover if I needed another dash into the trees, and I had little water left for the descent. Considering the rumbly state of my stomach, a need for discretion could be imminent. What if Justin made it to the top before me, then glanced down just to see me crouched on the side of the trail, emptying my sick bowels? I grimaced. *Not happening.*

Unbidden, I yawned again, my lips spreading so wide I thought my jaw would pop. Whatever lead I'd had would be gone by now. I struggled to keep my eyes open, too sleepy for panic anymore. All I wanted was a gallon of fresh water and a deep, dreamless nap.

I lay down under the last cluster of quaking aspens and stared up at the sky. Atticus lay down next to me, warm against my side. I burrowed the tips of my fingers into his hot fur.

"Just for a minute," I murmured through a yawn. The soft whisper of wind brushed my hair against my cheek. I snuggled my head against the pack and closed my eyes, willing my body to relax just a little.

Just for a few minutes.

The heady blackness of a deep nap stole over me, and I gladly welcomed it.

17

SOME PRIDE

When I woke up, something felt different.

My eyes flew open. Atticus stirred at my side, tilting his massive head back until it rested on my shoulders. The muscles in my arms and legs had the tight, stiff feeling of not having moved in hours. I blinked, staring at the sapphire sky. The numbers on my watch read 2:09.

I shot straight up.

We'd been asleep for hours.

My stomach gurgled when I leaped to my feet, and I instantly regretted my quick movement. The sore, inflamed muscles in my calves and thighs protested. I dropped back to the ground with a wince.

"The twins are going to kill me," I said to Atticus. "We were supposed to be back an hour ago."

Atticus hopped up—a bit more gingerly than usual—and wound his way through the aspens toward the trail.

Moving more slowly this time, I stood up. My head swam for a moment, then cleared. Nothing had changed in the landscape. The gentle breeze had faded. The sun had tracked farther against the sky. A brave ground squirrel chattered from behind a close rock. Despite my panic, I couldn't deny a sense of being physically rested, although my abdomen felt wrung out for an entirely different reason.

I paused, staring at the top of Custer Mountain. I'd been asleep for three hours, at least. I could still summit, but that would cost me time and energy. After my spectacular crash, I wasn't sure I had more ups and downs left to endure. What if the staff sent out a search party for me? I cringed at the thought.

Returning would be my best option, even though I had to face the ugly music: I owed Justin $500 I didn't have. The magic wand that was going to solve all my problems disappeared in a wisp of smoke. So much for the easy road out.

"Ugh," I groaned, kicking a rock. "The twins are never going to let me live this down."

Summiting Custer Mountain would have to come later. In the meantime, I had to figure out how to tell Justin I didn't have his money.

And get over the fact that I loathed biffies.

I STEPPED out of the biffy the next evening with a twisted face, my breath held. The heat of the summer had baked the small wooden house, turning the already sour air into something fetid. I hoped I could scrub the stench of urine off my skin.

"Looking good, Meg!"

"Is it just me, or is it definitely time for a little nap?"

A couple of staff strolled by, poorly attempting to cover their chuckles as they disappeared into the trees.

"Laugh it up," I muttered. "I'm fixing your dinner, and I just cleaned a nasty toilet, you overgrown children."

The skin of my fingers had wrinkled when I pulled my elbow-length plastic gloves off and tossed them into the bucket. Ten to go. Why did they have so many biffies? Couldn't the boys just pee in the trees? A second pair of feet approached me from behind, and I braced myself for another round of teasing.

"Whoa! Blister!" Mark waved a hand in front of his face. "Cut down on the fresh veggies, will you?"

I rolled my eyes.

"So." He waggled his eyebrows. "How's it going? Do you love your new job? Should I rearrange things so you can do this all the time? Or you can just take a nap if you're sleepy."

"Shut up."

He followed me as I moved past him, bucket in hand. Justin hadn't even gloated when I'd returned, metaphorical tail between my legs. Then again, by the time I reappeared exhausted, dehydrated, and wearing one shoe because I'd thrown the other into the trees in a fit of low-blood-sugar rage, pretty much everyone had been concerned. Thankfully, no one had brought up the exchange of money yet.

"JJ did try to warn you about the energy gels," Mark said. I strode down the trail so quickly that he moved into a slow trot. "I mean, to be fair. They're new and experimental, so obviously diarrhea would be an issue. And with that much caffeine, sugar, and ginseng?" He whistled. "You're lucky your blood sugar didn't crash into a coma."

"What do you want, Mark?" I snapped.

"Fine, fine. You don't have to worry about dinner tonight. JJ, Justin, and I have it covered."

I moaned. "That's even worse!"

He clapped me on the back. "Sometimes we fall so that we can get back up again."

"Get off me."

"Does it make you feel better if I point out that it will take three of us to replace you? And we're having JJ do his famous grilled cheese sandwiches. He claims he does it butter-free." His nose wrinkled. "We'll see how it pans out. He's coming out of veganism for this moment."

"He's vegetarian, Mark."

"Whatever."

I paused, considering. "Yes, it does make me feel a little better."

"Good." He pushed me back onto the trail. "Now go clean my biffies while I check on a possible bear sighting. Don't fall asleep!"

When I finished cleaning, I showered for twenty minutes with the hottest water I could tolerate, scrubbing my skin until it tingled. Although I hadn't enjoyed the process, I had *cleaned* those biffies.

Distant voices filled the background as I walked the trail from the outdoor staff showers, carrying my dirty clothes in a plastic sack. Darkness fell. The sunset faded between each tree, turning them into black spires. A nearby cricket chirped as I approached my cabin, grateful to be clean.

"Hey, Meg? Over here."

Although I couldn't see him, Justin's voice streamed through the trees by his cabin. The comforting scent of campfire lingered in the air. I dropped my bag in my cabin and headed over, my hair still damp on my shoulders. A fire flickered in a small stone circle, flaring toward the trees in orange and yellow tongues of flame. Justin sat with his back against a log. He motioned next to him with a tilt of his head.

"Have a seat." He nudged a plate covered with foil my direction. "I brought dinner for you."

"Is the kitchen closed?"

"They're running a big poker game." A brief lull in conversation brought a sound of guffawing from the lodge. "Thought this would be less chaotic."

I sat next to him, balancing the plate on my knees. "Thanks," I said. "That was really thoughtful of you."

He poked at the fire with a gnarled stick. The charred end sent a plume of red and orange sparks dancing into the air. I opened the foil to discover a grilled cheese sandwich and peeled orange slices. The tang of the juicy orange erased some of the bitter bleach taste in my mouth.

"This is delicious," I said, pulling off a piece of the sandwich. "JJ makes a mean grilled cheese."

We sat in the silence for several minutes after I finished eating. When I tossed the paper plate into the flames, the edges started to smoke and then curl. I watched it disintegrate into the crimson ashes and disappear amongst the coals, and then I pulled my knees into my chest and wrapped my arms around them. Justin looked over but said nothing.

"I have to admit something," I said, staring at the flames.

"Okay."

"I don't ... I don't have $500."

The fire glittered in his eyes when I met his gaze and quickly looked away.

"I made that bet because I'm a little behind on a credit card payment, and I really thought I could win. I'm sorry. I shouldn't have been so arrogant."

Desperate, I thought to add but clamped my mouth shut.

"You would have, I bet, if you hadn't crashed from those gels."

"Maybe," I murmured. "But that doesn't matter as much as the fact that I didn't win and I can't pay you right away. But I will! I *will* pay you. It just may take a few months."

"Meg, don't even worry about it."

"Of course I will. It's ... it's just embarrassing," I said into my jeans. "And it's even worse if you forgive it. I want to pay it. Just give me some time?"

He crossed his ankles and stuck his hands into his pockets. His casual, easy demeanor put me at ease. "Sure."

"Thanks."

"Did the bet have anything to do with your job search?" he asked. My shoulders tightened.

"Uh, yes. And no."

My mind felt like a sheet of black sandpaper. Gritty. Scratchy. Full of bumps. I didn't want to tell him the truth. I'm thousands of dollars in debt, have nothing but a return ticket home to my name, and don't know how I'll make it through the summer.

I couldn't ignore the thought fluttering around my head. *Justin has a lot of money. Maybe he could loan it to you.*

No. I shuddered. *I have* some *pride.*

"Want to talk about it?" he asked.

"Not really. But thanks."

"Anytime."

Atticus rolled onto his back, so I scrubbed his soft underbelly. The fire popped and crackled, casting Justin's eyes in deep shadow.

My thoughts unraveled. Jodie would call on Monday with job opportunities. With any luck, some of them would be open for the first of August, and I could sign a contract. It wouldn't pay my credit card on time, but I'd stay at Adventura and fulfill my promise to the twins. Whatever ripple effect occurred, I would deal with it then.

Going into debt had been my fault, not Mark and JJ's.

The sound of laughter rolled through the forest, washing over me. Having some kind of direction settled the lump in my chest.

Justin and I sat in the comfortable warmth of the campfire, so close I could feel the rise and fall of his chest. The scent of burning pine drifted through the air.

"You ready for a nap?" Justin asked, jarring me from my thoughts. "I mean, I can see you're getting comfortable and know you like taking siestas in the trees."

I shoved him in the shoulder with my own, failing to suppress a chuckle. His laugh rang out over the trees, banishing the sandpaper of my thoughts.

18

INADEQUATE

The seventh week of camp brought electric blue skies, marshmallow clouds, and the smell of sunscreen. Monday afternoon, I stepped out of my cabin after a short power nap and stretched my arms over my head with a yawn. A recipe for crazy milkshakes buzzed through my head. Chicken with ham and Swiss cheese would be the perfect complement.

"Hey, Meg," a voice called from behind me. "Is Atticus with you?"

Justin jogged up. Sweat streaked the sides of his face and neck, saturating his t-shirt collar. His breathing came in erratic bursts. He doubled over, mopping the perspiration from his face with the back of his arm.

"No," I said. "He sat with me at flag ceremony this morning, but I haven't seen him since. Everything okay?"

Justin's teeth sank into his bottom lip as he straightened, running a hand through his damp hair. He blew out a long breath. I tried to ignore the attractive elongation of his arm muscles. A light dusting of stubble shimmered on his jaw.

"I don't know," he said. "I don't think so. He's never been gone this long."

"How long?"

"Hours. Three. Maybe four? I was occupied dealing with a water issue at the main office and thought he was with JJ, but JJ hasn't seen him. I ran through all the campsites but found no sign of him."

The skin on the back of my neck prickled. Had he chased off a stray animal and lost his way back? Justin glanced over his shoulder as if expecting Atticus to trot up at any second. But a tense stillness descended on us instead.

Justin let out a long, controlled exhale. "I don't have a good feeling about this. Atticus doesn't just leave."

A buzzing sensation on my thigh interrupted my downward spiral. I pulled my phone out of my pocket to see Jodie Renner's name flash across the screen. My breath caught. Did she have a job for me? My thumb hesitated over the *answer* button before I shoved the phone back in my pocket. Jodie would have to wait.

"Let's spread out," I said. "We can cover twice the ground together."

He lifted his eyebrows. "You sure?"

"Of course. Where haven't you looked?"

"Thank you," he breathed. "Let's start at the river. He spends a lot of time there. I'll go west and follow it to the lake and around the back. You head east up the canyon. It's not likely he went that way. He never has."

I nodded. "You got it."

Justin strode off in the opposite direction while I slipped behind the lodge. The gentle whir of the rapids grew louder as I approached the busy stream. Water rushed over rocks and boulders, churning into white foam. Nothing unusual caught my eye. Several dog prints decorated the riverbank, but they could have been from this morning.

For fifteen minutes, I stuck close to the stream, wandering into the nearby glens of quaking aspens to shout Atticus's name. The happy shrieks and sounds of camp faded as I moved along. No sign of Atticus lingered in the dirt. My radio crackled on my hip.

"Justin for Meg, over."

"This is Meg."

"Anything?"

"No sign so far."

"Me neither. Sione and Hollis haven't seen him. I'm heading behind the lake. I'll keep searching south."

"You guys playing hide and seek with Atticus?" JJ asked. "I want in. Just finished at the wall. I'll ask at the rifle range."

Static overtook Justin's reply as I worked further upstream, ducking a low-lying branch covered with moss. A divot in the soft mud caught my eye. I crouched next to it.

"Grief," I muttered.

A perfect dinner-plate sized paw print of a bear was pressed into the soil. I bit my bottom lip and straightened. Maybe coming up the canyon alone hadn't been a good idea. An itch to return crawled down my back. A twig snapped. I whipped around as a squirrel scampered into the bracken with an annoyed chitter.

Imagining Atticus spending the night in the forest alone—if he was even out here—rallied my courage.

"Girl power, Meg," I said, rolling my shoulders. "Find Atty."

Despite my instinct to turn back, a niggling fear drove me on. I stepped on dried twigs, sang as loudly as I could, and veered away from the stream to call and listen. The lack of warbling birds made the forest feel naked and abandoned. On either side of the dense bushes, the canyon walls narrowed, growing steep and mossy beyond the scraggly pines. Boulder fields replaced the quaking aspens. My voice seemed to bounce off the rocks in an empty staccato. Thirty minutes of searching passed. I paused near a sapling, my boots soaked and calves flecked with mud.

It's not likely he went that way. He never has, Justin had said.

But what if?

With JJ, Justin, and possibly more of the staff searching by now, I could be spared to sneak a little further—just in case. The sun sank behind the crest of the mountain, coating the canyon in the first layer of early dusk. The radio static had faded into nothing; I'd hiked out of range. Another ten minutes passed. Disheartened, I let out a long sigh.

"You wouldn't come this far without a reason, Atty," I murmured, stepping on top of a fallen tree to better scan a clump of trees at the bottom of a steep, rocky pitch. "Now I'm just wasting time. They may have already found you."

Resigned, I turned to go, and an unusual pattern on the ground caught my eye. A paw print. I leaped off the tree. The circumference was too small to be a bear's but too big for a rodent's. My breath caught. Definitely canine.

The tracks moved away from the stream. I snaked alongside the slight indentations in the softened dirt with a hiccupping heart.

"Atticus," I called. "Atticus, come!"

A half-bark, half-whimper issued from beneath a rotting tree. I skirted around a clump of patchy evergreens. A black patch of fur lay on the ground. I fell to my knees with a cry.

"Atticus? Oh, Atty."

He lay on his right side, whining with every shallow exhale. Blood matted his ribs and belly where four slashes cut through the fur. Black puncture marks riddled his front leg like something had tried to break it. He licked his lips and tried to stand. A yip of pain stopped him. The dried blood on his fur meant hours must have passed. I reached out and put a soothing hand on his neck, pressing him down with a gentle hand. Crimson stained the rocks and soil beneath him.

"Whoa, boy. You're all right now. You're good. Just stay down." My eyes darted around. No sign of another creature, but the heavy vegetation near the stream could hide many dangers. "Let's get you home."

He calmed, laying his head back on the ground with a high-pitched cry. His eyes closed. I untied my jacket, draped it around his belly, hooked the radio to my neckline, and carefully grabbed him underneath his forelegs and hips.

"Nothing but a clean and press, Megan," I whispered, organizing my mind for a fluid, heavy lift. "Clean and press."

Atticus howled when I lifted him, ducked, and settled him on my shoulders in one seamless motion. My legs wobbled until I shifted his weight, finding my balance on the rocky terrain. He yipped and licked my hand, which held his back legs and uninjured foreleg in a firm vise.

"All right, buddy," I said. "Let's get you home."

The idea of an aggressive animal lingering in the thick shrubs pressed me hard back toward the stream. Once there, I waded into the water and started back. Navigating the edge of the stream, picking my footfalls amongst unsteady dirt and roots, would be impossible with eighty pounds of Atticus on my shoulders. Darkness fell fast in the high mountains.

It would be a long hike home.

Within minutes, my toes numbed in the icy water. Atty's blood, sticky and warm, soaked through the jacket and onto my neck. My arms, shoulders, and obliques smoldered like a bed of hot coals. Every time Atticus wriggled, the muscles in my hand cramped from holding so tight. I stumbled and fell to my knees often. My paranoia ran high—I studied every shifting shadow.

"Easy boy," I murmured, squatting to navigate a low-lying tree branch. The freezing water crept up my thighs. I clenched my teeth and sucked in a sharp breath. Every minute felt like a small eternity.

Slowly, the rocky terrain gave way to trees. The rush of the water slowed as the stream split into smaller gullies again. The radio picked up more static. A thread of JJ's voice came through the speaker.

"Meg? We are ... and ... where ... you?"

Releasing my hold on Atticus to answer would be dangerous for both of us, so I let JJ's voice continue, reassured that I was closing in on Adventura again. Atticus's weight intensified once he stopped fighting. Instead of trying to get away, he went limp on my shoulders.

I walked faster.

Twenty minutes later, a voice calling through the trees caught my ear. Atticus groaned but didn't stir. A familiar man bun popped into view ahead of us. I stopped mid-stride.

"JJ!" I cried. "We're over here."

"Meg! I've be—what the hell happened?" He reared back, eyes widening. Seconds later, he leaped into the stream and high-stepped toward us. "Tell me that's his blood and not yours."

"It's his."

"Let me take him."

"No! I'm not sure how bad his injuries are. The more he moves, the more he seems to bleed. He's calm. I can finish this."

JJ's eyes trailed to my shoulders. He nodded, lips pressed into a firm line. "Okay. I'll try to find a good path. Just follow me." He grabbed his radio and spoke into it. "This is JJ. Found Meg. She has Atticus. Meet us at medical."

"Roger," Justin replied. "Heading there now."

JJ and I waded out of the stream and onto the thin animal trail he'd been following. Stepping on solid ground with numb feet felt strange, like my feet didn't exist and only the hard bones of my leg remained. We burst into the medical cabin fifteen minutes later. It lay empty, though the sounds of campers echoed in the background. I carefully knelt while JJ threw a towel on the cot.

"Easy, pup," JJ crooned as he slid Atticus off my shoulders and straight onto the cot. I collapsed back, drawing in a deep, unburdened breath. Atticus released a pathetic bark, his eyes rolling. I scrambled back into action, put a hand on his head, and whispered until he calmed.

"We need to take him to a vet," JJ said. He reached down to help me up, his gaze lingering on my shoulders. "You look pretty intense, Meg."

When I reached to my neck, my hand came away smeared with blood. Despite the freezing stream, sweat trickled down my face and back. My fatigued muscles felt like Jell-O once they relaxed.

"Hold him there," I said. "Don't let him lick the wounds. I need to clean off the dried blood and see what we're dealing with."

JJ caressed Atticus's head while I grabbed a bottle of sterile water and ripped open a package of gauze. The cabin door slammed open. Justin tore inside, Mark on his heels.

"What happened?" Justin asked, rushing to the cot. JJ stepped back. Atticus lifted his head and whimpered, nuzzling his face into Justin's hand with a continuous, low cry in his throat.

"Meg found him up the canyon," JJ said. "Looks like he was attacked."

Mark clapped Justin on the shoulder. "I'll go for your Jeep, man. We need to get him into Jackson City. JJ, call Dr. Williams at the emergency vet clinic. Let her know we're coming."

While Mark and JJ bolted away, I draped soaked gauze across Atticus's wounds and slowly peeled the fur away. Justin swallowed, running his hand over Atticus's face in long, soothing strokes.

"How does it look?" he asked. I crouched next to the cot, dabbing carefully. The deepest wounds reflected a shining, crimson darkness. No sign of bone. No copious amount of blood to indicate that a major vein or artery had been damaged.

"I'm no dog expert ... but I think he'll be okay. Long recovery. Lots of stitches. But as long as nothing internal is going on, I'm hopeful."

Justin pressed his forehead against Atticus's and let out a long breath. I saturated more gauze and draped it over the wounds to cover them in the truck. Justin's eyes roved over me, lingering on my bloodied neck and shoulders.

"You're all right?" he asked.

"Yeah." I met his gaze for the first time. "I'm fine."

"Did you see what it was?"

My mind strayed back to the possible bear sighting that weekend. "No, but I think it was a bear. I saw some paw prints halfway to Atticus. Maybe he was chasing it off? He's probably a hero, preventing it from coming any closer."

He swallowed, nodding. The crunch of tires on gravel prevented further conversation. Mark leaped out of Justin's Jeep and pitched the keys to JJ, who was running back from the lodge where reception was best.

"Dr. Williams is expecting us," JJ said. "Let's go."

We wrapped Atticus in a thick blanket. Justin lifted him, cradling him in his arms as he slid into the back seat and set Atticus's head on his lap. Mark and I stepped back as the Jeep tore away in a cloud of dirt, JJ at the wheel.

Mark hooked an arm around my bloody shoulders and slapped me on the back. "Good work, little blister. And thanks."

I recoiled. "Why are *you* thanking me?"

Mark gazed at the haze of dust that lingered in the air. "Because you saved the dog, but you also saved the gladiator."

~

THAT EVENING, I snuck into Justin's cabin with a pile of old blankets and made a bed for Atticus on the floor. The tangy scent of aftershave with the lightest whiff of vetiver lingered in the air. My stomach fluttered. I left before I started snooping through his stuff.

Sleep remained elusive. Around ten, I slipped on my hiking boots and a warm jacket and trekked outside past the lodge. I caught sight of the distant flickers of dying campfires through the trees, accompanied by the sound of muffled laughter. The campers would be bedding down soon, and the world would descend into the tranquility of a mountain evening.

I turned onto the gravel road that led to the rifle ranges and walked halfway down it, then stopped. The sky unfurled like a bright canvas of glitter and velvet, filling the slot between the mountains with twinkling warmth. I stopped with a sigh and craned my head back until it hurt. Unable to tear myself away, I lay down on the road.

So wild. So untamed. Just like the mountain wilderness. I felt small beneath the blinking lights, and for a moment, it felt good just to be a part of something big.

My mind flashed back to Atticus and the fear in Justin's eyes—and then to Jodie Renner's missed call.

I gasped.

When I yanked my phone out of my pocket, only one bar of service came up. With any luck, I'd just be able to make out her message. I clicked through the phone to find two new voicemails. She must have called again.

"Megan, this is Jodie. Listen ... really good news ... found a flight position with a really ... hospital. New ... expanding ... There's a problem ... a ... hours away ... didn't know if ... move ... Need to know ... closes this evening. Call..."

I closed my eyes, already feeling the truth deep in my gut. Too late. But I sat up and clicked to the next voicemail anyway. This one came through with more clarity.

"Hey Megan, Jodie again. I waited late at work just in case you called, but I have to get to my son's basketball game. Sorry we missed this opportunity."

The distant edge in her voice didn't give me much hope for another chance. I deleted both voicemails and pushed the phone back into my pocket. Instead of bitter regret, a loose sense of relief and sadness tugged at me—I wouldn't go back and change anything. Atticus was alive and safe. What else mattered?

My thoughts fell into a whirling daydream of hanging out with Lexie again, having a boxing match with Traveler's Credit Card, and the punchy feeling in my gut when I saw Atticus lying on the rocky ground. His whimpers would haunt me all night long.

The sound of shifting gravel pulled me from my thoughts. When I tilted my head back, a broad-shouldered figure walked toward me, hands in his pockets. My stomach caught. Trailing ahead of him came the lightest hint of vetiver.

Justin stopped next to me, head tilted back to study the night canvas. I wondered if he'd ask why I was lying on a dirt road in the middle of the forest, then zipped my jacket the rest of the way when I realized I wasn't wearing a bra.

Again.

Instead of speaking, he lay down in the dirt next to me and stacked his hands behind his head. Just having him at my side felt natural. We stayed there for several minutes, staring at the stars in a long, comfortable silence.

"Atty okay?" I finally asked.

Justin readjusted his body. "Yes, thanks to you. He'll pull through. Required over thirty stitches, IV antibiotics, and pain medicine but should make a full recovery. No internal damage so far. High risk of infection. They put him under sedation while they cleaned him up, so he's still there. If the IV antibiotics work and he has no fever, he can come home in a few days."

I let out a long breath. "He's a tough pup."

Justin rubbed his weary face with a hand. "Yeah, he really is. I just keep thinking about how much worse it could be, and I'm glad this is all we have to deal with."

I studied him from the corner of my eye. The low light of the heavens threw sharp shadows on his cheeks, highlighting his dark stubble and long lashes. The ebbing pain I felt from losing the flight position disappeared completely. Jobs would come and go.

Justin turned to face me, startling me with the depth of his blue-gray eyes. "I don't know how to thank you, Meg. What if you hadn't kept going? We might have never found him. I don't ... I mean ... thank you. He's the only family I have left."

I swallowed. "I'm glad it worked out."

He opened his mouth to say something, stopped, and then said. "Yes, well, thank you, at any rate." He rolled his head back to face the stars, and I did the same, grateful for a little distance. "*Thank you* feels so inadequate when you saved his life."

"We all love Atticus. Any of us would have done the same."

His hand twitched at his side now. A steady chill lay like a blanket across the sleepy field, and I curled my fingers against my palm, surprised to find them cold. A yawn threatened my jaw. My thoughts had slowed to the sluggish pace of almost-sleep. The fading adrenaline of the day left me wiped out.

"Well," I said after another long silence. "I think I'm going to bed."

He stood up and offered me a hand. "I'll walk you back. I saw you walk out here just as I returned and came out to thank you and give you an update."

With a little smile, I accepted his hand, enjoying the warmth of his fingers pressed against mine before I pulled away. We trudged through the field. When we came to the split leading to our separate cabins, he stopped.

"Thanks again."

I smiled. "Anytime."

When I was only a few feet away from my cabin door, he called out. "Meg! Wait."

I spun around just as he strode up and scooped me into his arms, locking me against his chest. He felt wonderful. Powerful. Confident. His body sent fire through my skin. My heart pounded like a drum against my ribs, dizzy and bold. Could he feel it? Did he feel just as breathless?

"Thank you," he said against my shoulder. "Really."

He set me back down. I expected a sheepish smile, but he stared at me with a stormy, troubled gaze before he stepped back.

"Sleep well, Meg."

"Yeah," I whispered as he faded into the trees. My faint, "Goodnight," disappeared into the slumbering forest, leaving an empty maw behind.

~

Reasons Not to Like Justin

...

...

...

...

19

DEAD SERIOUS

Atticus returned to Adventura Friday afternoon to rampant applause from the staff. Sione draped a lei around his neck. Mark snuck him a three-ounce steak. And Justin fashioned a shirt to keep the dust out of his expansive wounds that said *Hero Dog of Adventura.*

Four puckered red lines studded with neat black stitches crossed a shaved patch of bare skin on Atticus's side. A white bandage twirled up his foreleg. He kept me company in the kitchen all day, settled on a comfortable bed of blankets arranged by JJ's detail-oriented eye. Atty's warm kisses felt better than any job offer.

~

"JJ," I said Sunday afternoon, "you may be able to climb almost any wall of rock known to man. You may have voted in more local elections than I have. And you carry the secret recipe for perfect vegan curry in your head and won't share, but that means nothing. I will beat you at The Game."

My fingers tapped the stack of cards lying in front of us. A resounding chorus of *ooh* sounded through the dining room. JJ's lips twitched.

"You boast a smooth play," he said, leaning back. His eyes tapered. "But my score is still tied with yours, which means you may not be the best anymore."

The muscles in my back cramped. I straightened, attempting to stretch them out. Vines of licorice, fun-size candy bars, and water bottles littered the table around us. To my right lay a pad of paper with two columns —*Megan: 190* and *JJ: 190*.

"Don't make a bet with her," someone called from the back. "She'll take a nap, and we won't get dinner!"

The staff jostled each other, guffawing under their breaths. I ignored them, keeping my eyes pinned on JJ. Flecks of gold ringed his hazel irises.

"You're determined?" he asked.

"You know I'm the master. No one's ever beaten me at The Game."

Hesitation flickered in his eyes. We'd played our family card game—a mixture of solitaire and pinochle—all night while camping as kids. The rules had formed in late nights of wild fatigue, eventually becoming a sacred tradition. The Game had always been in our lives.

And it had always been *mine*.

My fingers glided through the cards with smooth momentum, helping me rack up points my brothers couldn't match. Only JJ challenged me because he'd always stayed up late playing with me. Talking about boys. Basketball practice. Whatever came up.

He shuffled the cards, fanning a perfect bridge that made a *pfft* sound. Admittedly, his lack of acquiescence made me nervous. He couldn't care less about organized card games. Unlike Mark, JJ didn't thrive off competition unless it came from a rock. Which made his penchant for winning more aggravating. He tossed me the deck.

"Deal the cards. We'll see who's the family master."

The focused attention of the staff bore into my back. I couldn't fathom why they cared, but I surmised it had something to do with hope of JJ finally losing at something.

"Whoever wins walks away with eternal glory," I said. "The title may not, at any time, be revoked unless won back. Are you sure you're ready for this?"

He flicked his fingers.

"Deal the cards."

The cards darted out of my hand at expert speed. Not a single person spoke. Most of them had been following the challenge since it started early this morning. We'd recessed only for lunch. My head pounded. My eyes ached. I wanted to go for a run to clear all the sugar out of my system. But I stayed.

Today, honor was more important than health.

"All right, girl power," JJ drawled as he rearranged his handful of cards. "Get ready to lose your mind."

I studied my cards, mentally categorizing them before I committed to the speed portion of The Game. A promising hand. I could stack, rearrange. Make it work somehow. The high-pitched beep of my phone cut through the silent lodge. It sat on the table next to me, face up. When I reached for it, JJ shook a finger.

"No way. This is between you and me. A phone call can wait."

One word appeared at the top of my screen.

Blake.

I blinked. Blake? We hadn't spoken since I left West End and he couldn't hire me. My heart seized. I could think of only one reason Blake would call me on a random Saturday afternoon in the middle of July.

"JJ, I have to take it."

"Why?"

"It's important."

"Obviously. Tell me why."

"Play The Game already!" Sione called. "I'm not getting any younger."

A murmur of agreement rippled through the crowd. JJ grabbed his short stack, his hand poised to whip through it. It would start The Game, and I'd be obligated to play or lose. The third ring rippled through a tense silence. Voicemail would pick up soon.

"I can't tell you why it's important," I said, swallowing. "Just ... just trust me."

"It's Mark calling you, isn't it? You set it up to be a different name so you could somehow rig the deck." He leaned forward. "Nice try. Really. You almost had me there."

"Finish him off!" Sione raised his fist in the air. "Beat JJ. Beat JJ. Beat JJ."

The rest of the staff echoed the cry, stomping their feet and pounding their fists on the tables. My stomach twisted as the ringing stopped. Despite the ruckus, the room felt empty without the phone warbling. My tense shoulders eased, although my mind wouldn't stop spinning.

Could Blake hire me?

"Pick up your cards." JJ nodded toward my pile. "Let's finish this off."

My hand trembled as it hovered over the deck. The phone beeped. *A voicemail.* I itched to answer but turned my attention to The Game. *You can do this, Meg,* I thought. *Just focus.* Ten more minutes of playing and I'd secure my victory. Then I'd call Blake back.

I dropped a heavy hand on the deck.

"Begin."

The cards flew out of our hands. I stacked, moved, arranged, and watched the cards disappear onto the table, racking up points. Every card mattered. Five minutes into the hand, we hit a plateau. JJ's eyes flicked from my hand to his as he moved through his deck. I bit my bottom lip. There had to be *something*. I had one card left. Victory was—

My phone buzzed with a text.

A message flashed across the screen. *Call me ASAP.* For a second, my life hung suspended in the balance. Adventura seemed to pause. I thought of work. Of late nights. Early mornings. Doctors. Alcohol swabs. Feeling good about myself at the end of a shift. *August 10th.* Credit card collection phone calls. The sweet little townhouse I'd purchased last fall.

With a sigh, I turned my whole attention back to The Game.

One minute later, the stalemate ended when I tossed down a seven of diamonds. With two lightning-quick moves, I closed The Game. JJ leaned back, sucking on his teeth. We still had to tally the points. If JJ had thrown out more cards than me, he could still win. My heart pounded.

"Ready, Megara?" JJ asked, eyes glimmering.

"Are you?"

The staff seemed to be holding their breaths as we separated the cards. To secure the win, we both counted our stacks out loud.

"Twenty-five," JJ said, smirking. "Beat that."

Respectable. I'd have to have twenty-six. My fingers whirred through the cards as the staff counted out loud as one. When I neared twenty, I felt my pile thinning down. Would it be enough?

"Twenty-three ... twenty-four ... twenty-five ... twenty-six!"

My hands raised in victory, and a wild cry erupted from the staff. Sione banged the table with his fists. Mark recorded the moment on his phone. In the background, someone cracked open a bottle of sparkling cider. JJ grinned, a lopsided smile on his face.

"I concede the crown is yours." He held up his hands. "You are the Master of The Game."

"Thanks!" I said, wrapping him in a hug. Then I threw down my cards, snatched the phone from the table, and disappeared outside, leaving the celebration behind me.

~

MY FEET SEEMED to be tied together as I scurried away from the lodge, the call ringing in my ear. I found my footing and speed-walked to my cabin. The quiet of the forest struck me as odd after the hours of excited noise. Seconds later, I heard Blake's voice crackling through the phone.

"Meg?"

"Hey, Blake," I said with forced ease, clutching the phone with white-knuckled fingers. "Can you hear me?"

"A little distant, but yeah. I can make you out."

"Good! Sorry I missed your call, but I just got your text." I swallowed the heavy lump in my throat, affecting the best nonchalance I could manage. "What's up?"

"Feels like it's been forever since you were poking around work, trying to find a job like a lost puppy." He chortled.

"Ha," I said with a little laugh. "You miss it. Is that why you're calling? Do you have a job for me?"

As if I *actually* felt so nonchalant about it.

"Yes, actually," he said. "If you want it."

The world stopped spinning. All my concentration focused on those words. This couldn't be real. Not mere days after losing the other position. Not at West End. At *home*. Where everything could tie up in a big, fat bow and fit together so nicely.

"Seriously?" I asked.

"Yep."

"In the flight department?"

"Well, I'm certainly not about to hire you for the pediatric unit."

I sank to the edge of my bed, my knees weak. Although I'd spent the last fifteen minutes hoping his phone call *would* mean this, I could hardly believe it. Return to all the people I knew at West End? Work on the helicopter? Achieve all my goals? And make great money in the meantime? I leaped to my feet to pace across the cabin. Nothing came this easy. There had to be a catch.

"I'm intrigued. Tell me more," I said.

"One of our guys was injured in a car accident and will be out. Possibly for a long time. We need someone to fill his spot immediately."

The list of other qualified applicants at West End ran through my mind. Blake had half a dozen other nurses that had salivated over the job just like me, all of them internal. Would I even have a chance? My hope faded. This hadn't been about a job after all. He just wanted me to apply.

"And you want me to apply?" I asked, my shoulders slumping.

"Nope. I want to hire you."

"But ... I thought..."

"That I couldn't hire you because you're an outside hire?"

"Yes."

"I pulled some strings and called in some favors. You know I wouldn't work on a weekend if I didn't have to. This would help me out a lot. I can't pull from other units on such short notice—not with a staffing shortage like this."

My breath caught. How could I say no? "You're serious about this, Blake?"

"Dead serious."

"When do you need me?"

"Today. Tomorrow. Monday at the latest. We have to get you trained and ready to go, so we'll be tight with staffing in the meantime."

My eyes screwed shut. I balled my hands into a fist. *No. No. No. This isn't happening!*

I cleared my throat. "Uh ... that may be a small problem. I'm not in town. And I can't just leave right now."

"Where are you?"

"In the mountains. I'm working for my brother this summer as the camp nurse and chef."

Blake blew out a heavy breath. "Okay, well ... when can you be here? Like two days?"

"The ninth of August."

"That's weeks away!"

The flame of hope flickered a little. I swallowed. "I know. There's still three weeks of camp left."

"And you can't leave?"

"Well ... no."

"What would happen if you did?"

What *would* happen if I left Adventura? Would they have to close it down? Mom could be a nurse here for a few weeks, I imagined. Couldn't she? Or Mark could call one of his thousands of friends to fill in, surely. It didn't even have to be a nurse. An EMT. A paramedic. Anyone with a pulse and a certification or license could do this job.

"I'm not sure," I said.

An awkward tension rose between us.

"Listen, Meg, this is a big deal. I *need* you."

Anxiety surged through my chest, making it difficult to breathe. "I know, Blake. I appreciate it. It's just—can I have some time to think about it? How long until you need an answer?"

"Oookay. Tomorrow, I guess? I can give you twenty-four hours to decide. Not a minute later. If I don't hear from you by 4:30 tomorrow, I'm going to my number two."

"Okay. Okay, great. I'll have an answer for you by then. Thank you so much."

My nails bit into my palm when I gripped a handful of hair in my fist and closed my eyes, praying he didn't tell me to stuff it and hang up. The pause that ensued grated on my nerves. I wanted to reach through the phone and shake him.

"Megan, I get that extenuating circumstances are at work here, but I put a lot of footwork into this approval. If you can't make it happen..."

His trailing pause froze my heart into a ball of ice. Would failing to accept break ties permanently with the West End Flight Team? Blake and his crew were my people. We had pumped chests and saved lives together in the CICU already. Working with them as an actual flight colleague would mean everything to me.

"Got it," I said. "Thanks, Blake."

He hung up after a curt farewell. I let the phone drop to my sleeping bag as I buried my face in my pillow.

What was I going to do?

Flight Job Pros List

- *$$$*
- *Won't have to move.*
- *Wear a jumpsuit. (Basically an adult onesie)*
- *Meet every goal I made in college.*
- *Near the Health and Happiness Society again.*
- *Buy a new car with working A/C.*
- *Work with West End Flight Team.*
- *Awesome resume.*
- *Continue my yoga classes with Bitsy.*

Flight Job Cons List

- *Mark will hate me.*
- *JJ will be disappointed in me.*
- *Parents have issues*
- *Adventura will suffer.*
- *Miss Atticus. Ok. Justin too*
- *I won't like myself.*

20

FOR THE BEST

The staff stayed away from the kitchen that evening, as if they sensed the bellow of my internal dragon. I dumped ingredients together for Leftover Soup, slapped butter on slices of French bread, slung it into the oven, and told JJ to pull it out in ten minutes. While the staff ate, I shoved a paddle board out onto the lake and stayed there until dark descended.

In desperation, I tried calling Mom once I got back to my cabin. She would loan me some money just to get me through August—even though bringing this up at a time when her marriage was struggling felt trite. But she didn't answer, even though I called three times. Finally desperate, I tried calling Dad, but his phone went right to voicemail. Livid, I tossed the phone across the room and stared at the ceiling.

Every hour crawled by with irrepressible leisure that night, one minute ticking into the next until I could hardly stand it. My mind whirred with the ugly truth—no matter what I chose, something would suffer.

Dad's distress in the restaurant bounced around my head. Mom's swollen, bleary eyes. The pain of their discord struck a deep note that resonated into my bones. Such disharmony had been avoidable, surely. People mattered more than careers or accolades or job offers. Mark, JJ, the staff, even Atticus—they meant more to me than anything.

Which meant I shouldn't take the job.

But determination, sacrifice, and talent had fueled my impressive career. Adventura would end soon. My life—my need for a job—wouldn't. My mind spun through all the people I'd helped, the lessons I'd learned, the families I'd met, all in the pursuit of something good. I *belonged* in the hospital. Besides, this flight-nurse opportunity would solve my debt issues. No creditors calling. No further marks on my credit to hurt me in the future. No loss of car or home. Mark and JJ would understand.

I should definitely take the job.

Finally, at three in the morning, I fell into a restless sleep. A syringe and stethoscope chased me in my dreams. I ran but barely stayed ahead of the gleaming needle. Just when I thought I'd escaped it, Blake blocked my path, despondent. I skidded to a stop, but the needle slid into my back, right near my heart.

A heavy thud on my door woke me at six the next morning. I jerked awake, nearly falling off the narrow cot.

"Up, blister," Mark called. "Campers arrive soon."

Yawning, I crawled out of my sleeping bag. I still had ten hours to make my decision.

Tick, tick, tick.

~

THAT AFTERNOON, dust billowed around the broom as I swept dirt from the lodge floor into the fireplace. Most of Adventura lay quiet and empty except for the occasional shout from the campsites, where the campers were eating lunch. The clock ticked in the background.

Decide. Decide. Decide, it seemed to say.

I can't. I can't. I can't.

The radio attached to my hip crackled seconds before Mark spoke. "Hey, Megan. Can you come out to the rifle range?"

I paused mid-sweep. The rifle range? Images of bullet holes and bloody limbs drifted through my mind. No one should be out there right now.

"Uh, sure. Everything okay?"

"Soon as possible."

"Injury?"

"No."

I propped the broom against the wall and left, enjoying the sunshine as I rambled down the two-track road out to the rifle range. Every now and then the *boom* of a shotgun rolled over the open range. Dad's old Chevy caught my eye, parked just outside. My heart leaped into my throat. I jogged the rest of the way.

"Hey," I said, a little breathless. "I'm here."

JJ leaned against the rifle range wall behind the gun tables, arms folded across his chest. He'd never been a big fan of firearms. No one spoke. Dad reloaded in his usual record time, glancing over his shoulder to me with a nod before resuming his concentration. After his final round—right in the bullseye—he lowered the rifle to his side.

"What are you doing here?" I asked him.

Dad loaded two slugs into a nearby shotgun, pressed it to his shoulder, peered down the barrel, and closed one eye. "In the area. Thought I'd stop by. Your mom is on her way."

With his foot, he tapped a clay pigeon machine. An orange disk hurtled into the air. Dad pulled the trigger, and the flying clay disk exploded. Everything about this felt weird. JJ's averted gaze. Dad's focused attention. Mark's tense jaw. The strangely calm scene sent me into a vortex of panic. Why weren't Mark and Dad arguing? They always argued. Even in jest.

Why was Mom coming while Dad was here?

JJ lounged back, eyes on the horizon, as if he were somewhere else. The rigid lines of his body had tightened. Mark's brow furrowed in a heavy bank over his eyes. I pressed a hand to my stomach, feeling sick.

Moments later, Mark grabbed a handgun, loaded three clips, and proceeded to unload them as fast as he could into the closest target. The *ping* of the falling shells echoed in the range. I stood next to JJ. He leaned against me until our shoulders touched, and I welcomed his steady, warm reassurance. No one spoke. Communication seemed like more than any of us could bear in such a looming quiet.

Fifteen minutes later, Mom's SUV tore up the road, a cloud of dust billowing around it. Dad loaded the gun and prepared to shoot again.

Like a scene from a movie, Mom's car rolled to a stop. The car door closed. Her feet ground on the loose gravel, and then she stood there wearing sunglasses. Her short-cropped hair shifted in the wind.

"Hey," Mom said, forcing a bright tone. She didn't take her sunglasses off. "Thanks for, uh, meeting your father and I here. I don't have long. I have to head to work."

Mark emptied a fourth clip, cleared the gun, and set it down on the counter. When he turned around, his eyes had hardened into circles of steel. JJ straightened. His shirt whipped in the wind. I wanted to hide behind him. Mom shifted.

"Just say it," Mark said, breaking the interminable silence.

The corners of Mom's lips turned down. She reached for him, but he stepped back and nearly ran into me.

"Mark, honey—"

"Say it!"

Dad stood several feet away from Mom, hands on his hips, looking at no one. That's when I knew. That's when I saw the dark shape that had been standing between all of us. They'd come to tell us the bad news—this was the end for my parents.

I sank. Down, down, down. Into the murky depths of disbelief, where the truth waved around me like faint ripples of light from far above. All I had to do was reach out and touch it. But when I did, it shimmered away without substance.

"Jim," Mom said, motioning to us as a group. Her voice caught. "Why don't you go ahead and tell them?"

He cleared his throat.

"No secret there's been problems," he said. "No reason to beat around the bush either."

Next to me, JJ tensed. I reached over and grabbed his hand. He squeezed my fingers. Mark's hands tightened into fists at his side. Dad looked up, peering at us from underneath the brim of his hat.

"We're divorcing," he said. "We feel it's for the best. We love you kids. More than anything, of course. That will never change. But it's time for Kelly and I to move forward, and we've realized we can't do that together."

Mom showed no visible reaction. For the span of a full minute, only the wind brushed past us in the background. My hair bounced behind me, trailing in long brown strands. Dad licked his lips, his gaze on the ground. A tear trickled down Mom's cheek and dropped onto her shirt.

Words threatened to pour out of me, but I swallowed them back. They clogged my throat like a heavy stone. Had I been wrong to hope? Had the writing been on the wall the whole time, and I just hadn't seen it?

Mark's feet shuffled against the dirt, drawing our attention. "Thanks for letting us know," he said, his voice cold with cordiality. "But I need to go finish a few things. So do they. It's a work day."

Mom reached for him again. "Mark," she murmured, but he moved away, stepping out of her reach. He disappeared down the road, striding with a long gait. JJ pushed away from the wall, and without looking to either parent, followed Mark. Mom and Dad's stares landed on me.

"Meg," Mom said. This time, she didn't reach out. "We're so sorry."

Panic welled up in me, hot and fast. *Stop!* I wanted to scream. *Stop acting so calm when everything is falling apart!*

My voice spoke, but I didn't recognize it as my own.

"I know."

Dad kicked a rock with the tip of his cowboy boot. "Has nothing to do with you." For a brief moment, his eyes met Mom's. They both looked away.

"We should have waited, Jim," Mom said under her breath. "I told you we should have waited until the end of the summer."

"They would have been just as upset then."

"Mark has a camp to run!" Mom snapped, whirling around to face him. "And now we've just broken his heart."

Dad's nostrils flared. "He would have been more upset if we'd waited until it was final. He's a man. He can handle bad news like a man."

Mom scoffed, a tinge of wild hysteria in her voice. "Right. That's rich coming from you."

My head collected their words like a butterfly net. They bounced around in a whirl of confusion. Then the wind tunnel that blew through my mind obscured their voices. Spittle flew from Dad's mouth as he countered a rebuff from Mom, who gesticulated with her hands. I covered my ears.

"Stop!" I screamed. "Just *stop*!"

The wild echoes ceased when they both turned to stare at me. Tears trickled down my cheeks, but I didn't know when they'd gotten there.

"Don't you see that I'm right here?" I thumped my fist on my chest. "This isn't just about *you*, you know. You're tearing apart our family, and now you're fighting in front of me like a bunch of twelve-year-olds."

Both of their faces dropped. Another tear fell down Mom's cheek from behind her sunglasses. "Meg." She stepped toward me. Like Mark, I retreated.

"Dad." I wheeled around to face him. "You ignored me when I tried to apologize and haven't come by until now. And Mom, you're running away to work and ignoring us. We've hardly seen either one of you all summer. You say it's not about us? You're right. Nothing is about us anymore. It's about you and your problems and your avoidance of your problems."

I scrubbed the tears off my cheek with the back of my arm, sniffling.

"I'm sorry this happened," I said, teary. "I really am. My heart breaks for all of us. But I ... I need time to think and ... I'm leaving."

The moment I said the words, the decision cemented in my heart. *Yes,* I thought in relief. *Home. To flight nursing.*

Mom's eyes widened.

"I just landed a job as a flight-nurse at West End. Nathan broke up with me the week before I flew out here. The next morning, I was laid off. I'm in debt. So badly in debt that I literally have no money in my bank account, and creditors are calling me. I have to have money by August tenth, and I just received an offer, so I'm taking the job."

Releasing the weights that had been pressing on my shoulders felt like flying. Why hadn't I done this sooner? The euphoria almost erased the pain. Almost helped me forget the strangling feeling of not knowing what to say.

Mom's mouth worked up and down. Dad's eyes tapered.

"Meg, why didn't you say something?" Mom whispered.

Tears filled my eyes.

"I tried. I called. I even kept your secret. But when could I have asked you for help? When was it ever about us and not the two of you?"

Dad closed his eyes. Unable to bear it, I shuffled back. "I'm sorry," I whispered. "But I have to go."

~

WITH TEARS STREAMING DOWN my face, I yanked my duffel out from underneath my cot and shoved clothes inside. If I slowed my momentum at all, I'd question everything. I had to go. The light in the cabin dimmed. JJ stood in my doorway, leaning one shoulder against the wood. He watched my panicked movements for almost a full minute before he broke the silence.

"You're going back?" he asked.

"I have a job offer for a flight-nurse position," I said. Tears blurred my vision. My lip trembled. "That's the call I received yesterday. I'm over two thousand dollars in debt to a credit card company and have no money. The new job needs me immediately. I'm going to call my friend Rachelle, beg her to put money in my bank account, then go to the airport and change my flight to this evening."

His jaw tightened. JJ's touch-oriented nature and natural compassion made him the most understanding person in our family—but also the most sensitive. Unfortunately, I had already passed the point of no return. I closed my heart off to the whispers of doubt and kept going forward.

"Why didn't you tell us you were having money problems?" he asked.

I chuckled without humor, shaking my head. "Were you going to loan me the money? Adventura has you farther in debt than I am."

His silence responded for him.

"Are you really leaving because of the job?" he asked. "Or is this about Mom and Dad? Mark and I are upset too. We—"

"How can they do this, JJ?" I asked, fixated on the way my fingers were shaking. "How can they just give up on each other?"

His shoulders slumped. "I don't know."

"I can't stay. I-I can't."

Something passed between us that tied my stomach in knots. Everything seemed to shake, although nothing moved.

The strap of the duffel bag bit into my shoulder when I jerked it off the cot and set it on the floor. I grabbed my backpack next and tossed my toiletries inside. Random belongings still littered the cabin. Old sneakers that needed to be thrown away. A half-eaten protein bar. Two mismatched socks that hung from the window ledge. I'd miss this musty, cold place.

Once I finished, I slung the backpack over my shoulder and grabbed the duffel. "Do you remember the day we went climbing when camp first started?" JJ asked. "I told you I was worried about Mom and Dad. You lied to me, didn't you?"

His words sent me into a panic spiral. The edges of my nails dug into my palms. I licked my lips, my mouth dry.

"I didn't lie."

"But you didn't tell me the truth. Isn't that a lie?"

The gentle, even cadence of his voice gave him away. This had been a surprise for JJ. Maybe not a *total* shock; he'd known something was going on. But if the betrayal and pain in his eyes meant anything, Mom and Dad hadn't included him in any of their sordid updates.

And neither had I.

"JJ, I promised Mom—"

"That you wouldn't tell me anything? Give me a damn heads-up?" He shook his head with a bitter hiss. "You also promised that I'd always have you to rely on. That even if something bad happened with Mom and Dad, we could still be a family."

JJ glanced down at my bag.

"Sure looks like it," he said. "Doesn't it?"

Twenty seconds passed before I could wrestle beyond my pain well enough to speak. "JJ, I can't stay. I'm sorry that you feel betrayed, but so do I. And you're right. I should have told you, but I had also promised Mom I wouldn't. And I … I didn't want it to be real. Like a fool, I believed they'd work through it."

The words fell from my lips like a dying wind.

"Mark is out on the trails," he said, pulling in a deep breath. "He's cleaning up the campsites, but I suspect he's really just burning off some energy. You need to at least talk to him before you go."

"I can't." My voice caught on the words. Facing Mark would destroy my dwindling resolve. I'd see in his eyes what my departure would mean. Perhaps I already knew what would happen if the only licensed medical person left.

"Can't?" he asked. "Or won't?"

A thick lump rose in my throat.

"Both."

He shook his head, his jaw tight. Tears welled up in my eyes. "I'm sorry, JJ," I whispered. "I have to go."

He didn't move as I shuffled past him and ran out the door as fast as I could, a sob blocking my throat.

~

Megan: Blake, I'm in. I want the job.

Blake: Awesome! Can you be here ASAP?

Megan: Just got a ride to the airport and my flight switched to today. I will be there tomorrow morning.

Blake: See you then.

21

IT'S MY WORD

The humid summer air nearly choked me when I returned home that evening.

The moment I stepped out of the airport and into the thick heat, I missed the dry scent of evergreen. City lights dotted the landscape. Even the whir of cars whizzing by felt out of place. I'd only been at Adventura for seven weeks, but it felt like a lifetime.

"I grabbed a pizza for dinner," Rachelle said as she pulled into traffic. "Let's just go to your house and ... uh ... sort things out."

I sank lower into the seat.

"Thanks."

Rachelle sent uncertain glances my way the whole ride home. We didn't speak. I didn't want to talk about it. She must have had so many questions —why didn't I call Lexie? Why was I back early? Why did I need to borrow money? But she asked nothing. Which was precisely why I'd called her.

We're divorcing. I kept hearing my dad's voice in a loop in my head. *It's for the best.*

An hour later, the door to my townhouse squeaked open. After weeks, the air smelled musty and old. Everything remained where I'd left it, though a light layer of dust coated the house. Rachelle flipped on the lights while I dropped my bags, advancing farther into the room.

"I should have come over and opened it up before your flight came in," she said, her nose wrinkling.

I waved it off. Remnants of everything I'd left behind cluttered my table and counters. An old headlamp that didn't work. A dirty pair of jeans. My stethoscope draped over the back of a kitchen chair. I walked past it without touching it.

"So," Rachelle said, following me into the kitchen, tossing the pizza box on the table. She wore a pair of jeans and a *Walking Dead* t-shirt. "Do you want to talk about what happened?"

"Not really."

"Too bad. We're going to talk anyway." She flipped open the pizza box and sank her teeth into a slice with a light moan. "OMG," she groaned. "I've missed this. Just ... don't tell Bitsy, okay?"

I grabbed the teakettle and pushed it under the water spout. The stream of water sputtered for a second before flowing free. Telling her about my cowardly exit—and the demise of my parents' marriage—would force me to relive all the pain and shame. Not something I felt inclined toward. But Rachelle had lived through her parents divorcing. Another of the many reasons I'd called her instead of Lexie.

For some reason, I just couldn't face Lexie right now.

Rachelle sobered as I sat next to her at the white wooden table, sinking into the chair as if I hadn't sat in days.

"Out with it, Megan Bailey." She slid a slice my way. "I want to hear everything."

I pulled in a deep breath.

"Okay."

I told her everything, starting with the night Nathan broke up with me, through the job loss, the creditors calling, all the way up to Blake's phone call offering me the job. Piece by piece, she listened to my life review, murmuring in all the right places. But still, my heart ached.

Rachelle leaned back. "Sucks, doesn't it? Divorce is the worst."

Exhausted, I slumped in my seat, rubbing a hand over my eyes. My second cup of tea had turned cold.

"I know."

She leaned forward, her earlobes glittering with sparkly black earrings.

She'd lost more weight in the past six weeks. I almost hadn't recognized her at first.

"So?" she asked. "What are you going to do?"

"Work. I start tomorrow morning. Then I can pay off my debt in time, keep myself out of credit hell, and figure out how to deal with this whole divorce thing in the meantime."

Unable to meet her gaze, I dunked my teabag up and down in the tepid water. While my townhouse held all my belongings, it didn't feel familiar anymore. I felt like a stranger in a strange land. The kitchen here seemed too neat, as if it had been put together for a magazine photo shoot. The flawless stovetop hadn't ever met three pans of spaghetti sauce. I didn't even know how the oven baked a loaf of homemade bread.

My heart sank a little deeper in my chest.

This place was supposed to be home. I remembered the ratty, poorly lit kitchen at Adventura. The deep laughter of the staff rolled through my mind. No one would walk through here and try to spray me with the sink nozzle. Or un-alphabetize the pantry while I wasn't looking. The closeness of the walls felt suffocating after I'd lived under a wide expanse of stars and mountains. The warmth of Adventura seemed suddenly more permeating than anything I felt here.

Chills brushed me, and I shuddered.

"Do you remember your parents' divorce?" I asked, needing the spotlight off myself. Maybe Rachelle could shed a little light into my all-encompassing darkness.

Rachelle leaned back against her chair with a heavy sigh. "A little. I was pretty young at the time. I remember being confused. Having nightmares. Feeling scared at night. Not much else. There's a sense of betrayal, I think, no matter when it happens. Nothing makes it better, either."

Her solidarity comforted me.

"I came back because life here used to make sense." My eyes darted over the too-small walls. "I was hoping it would make sense now."

She glanced around, and I wondered what she saw. "Does it?"

"No."

"Are you expecting it to?"

"Hoping, more like it." I swallowed. "I don't think it ever will again."

Rachelle rolled her lips together. "No," she whispered. "For a while, it won't. And even then, it'll be a whole new kind of normal. Holidays, birthdays, all that will be different."

Tears filled my eyes. I downed the last of the cold tea and set the cup back down. A heavy ball of agitation had been unrolling in my chest ever since the plane landed. It threatened to break free. Taking my heart and all its many broken pieces as its victim.

Rachelle stood up.

"I'll give you some space," she said. "I recognize that look. Call me, okay, if you just need to talk."

I cleared my throat.

"Yeah. Will do." My voice deepened with emotion, grateful to be left alone with my thoughts. "Thank you, Rachelle."

THE NEXT MORNING, I stared at the golden plaque on Blake's door. My heart beat a heavy staccato beneath my ribs. Every time I blinked, sandpaper moved under my eyelids. Sleep hadn't come easily, despite a king-sized bed all to myself. Behind me, two staff members walked by, the lines in their faces deep, their gait slow.

Brushing it off, I squared my shoulders and stared at Blake's name again. *Focus, Megan,* I thought. *This means everything.*

With a sigh, I reached up with a fist to rap on the door, but a buzz from my phone caught my attention. I'd been avoiding all phone calls since leaving Adventura. Mom had called five times last night before I silenced it. With a rush of courage, I checked the screen.

Voicemail (2)

Jodie Renner

I tucked it back into my pocket. I'd call her after I spoke with Blake. My knuckles rapped quietly on the door. Seconds later, the door swung open. Blake grinned, a toothy smile on his stubbled, thin face. He stretched an arm into his office, which overlooked the landing pad through sprawling glass windows.

"Megan Bailey," he said. "Welcome home."

With a relieved sigh, I stepped into his office.

Organized stacks of paperwork littered his mahogany desk. Two young girls smiled from his computer screen. He wore a pair of scrub pants and a t-shirt, and his badge jangled with every movement. I missed the singsong of hospital life. The overhead paging system. Phones ringing. Medication drawers slamming. Being back inside reaffirmed what I already knew deep in my bones: I belonged in a hospital.

Outside, the blades of the helicopter spun so fast they appeared not to move at all. A nurse ran out in a flight suit, leaping inside. The door closed behind her.

My stomach clenched.

That will be me soon.

The thrill I'd expected didn't come. Instead, I pictured Mark sitting on the counter at Adventura, his heels banging into the cupboard as he told me about his day and laughed at his own terrible jokes. Blinking, I cleared the picture from my mind and sat down.

Maybe the jokes hadn't been that terrible.

"So," Blake drawled. "How does it feel being back?"

I smiled, forcing it wider. "Awesome. I think West End missed me."

He snorted. "Confident. I like it."

"How are things going here?" I asked. "With the hiring freeze and cutbacks?"

He shrugged but didn't make eye contact. "You know. It's going. A lot of people were understandably upset. Budgets are a little tight. But thankfully we're making it work. Next to your impressive resume, I think that's the reason they approved your hire, to be honest. You worked for us so recently, it'll save money."

Way to sweep me off my feet, West End. But what did it matter? At least I had the job. Even if my home felt strange, my best friend was getting married, and my parents were divorcing, I always had my career.

"And the CICU?" I asked. I pictured Karen's haggard face. "How are things going down there?"

"Fine."

He leaned forward, flapping a hand.

"Enough of that stuff. Let's get down to business. You'll sign the contract with Michelle in HR, but I like to meet with new hires and discuss the training schedule, expectations, etc."

He grabbed a folder and flipped it open, producing a thick wad of papers that he tossed to me. They landed with a light *thump*. The professional header across the top made my heart flutter.

West End Flight Team.

Swallowing back a swell of emotion, I scanned the words that directed the next step in my career. Phrases jumped out at me. *Full-time position. Twenty-four hour shifts. Training modules completed to success. OR rotations. Survival training.*

Although Blake said something every now and then, I felt as if I were alone in a vacuum of silent words and the ghosts of my decisions. Why did my hands feel clammy? Why couldn't I focus on the words? The whole paper seemed to blur in front of me. I re-read the third line four times before moving on, having no idea what it said.

"—starting immediately. I'm really excited to have you on our team, and so is everyone else. Although you've only worked here a year, everyone speaks very highly of you—"

Besides, I wouldn't even make you sign a contract, Mark said in the back of my mind, overriding Blake's easy chatter. *That's how much I trust you, blister.*

Like a landslide overwhelming my heart, the truth fought a mighty battle against my walls. And won.

I never should have left Adventura.

Mark's words swept over me again and again, circling back to the ugly arithmetic. I'd abandoned my brothers. My Adventura family. Justin. Sione. Hollis. For the first time, I allowed myself to ask: What *would* happen in my absence?

And why hadn't I asked that before I left?

Tears filled my eyes from a deep, aching remorse. What had I done? Blake shouldn't hire me. Not because I wasn't qualified but because I wasn't honest. This wasn't *right*.

"Meg?"

I jerked out of my reverie. Blake peered at me.

"You all right?"

"Oh, sorry." I rubbed a hand over my face. "Yes. I just ... I just lost my train of thought. Sorry."

He lifted an eyebrow. "Okay. Well, like I said, the work agreement extends out for—"

"Blake, wait. I have to stop you there."

He snapped his mouth shut and raised his eyebrows. "Yes?"

I swallowed.

"Listen, I'm sorry. But..." I slid the sheaf of papers back to him. His brow lowered. "I can't take this job."

My fingers braided together in a knot of ice on my lap. I squeezed them so tight my nails blanched white. *Don't do this!* my mind screamed. *You're giving up a golden opportunity.*

No, I said, responding to my own inner fear. *This is the right thing to do.*

Blake frowned. "I'm sorry. You ... can't?"

"No."

"Do you mind if I ask why?"

My shoulders lifted as I drew in a deep breath. "Because I wasn't honest in how I came to this job. I-I mean that I was working somewhere else this summer, and I just left them. In a big lurch, I think. I *want* to work for you. But ... it wouldn't be the right thing to do." I bit my bottom lip. "Besides, things aren't good in my family right now. I'd like to be close to them. I can't do that here."

Blake leaned back in his chair. "What did you do there? Throw together some sandwiches and bandage knees? This is real life stuff. You're turning down a major promotion and a salary increase. I mean, c'mon, Meg. It's a summer camp."

"No." I shook my head. "It's my word."

He spread his arms. "But you've wanted this job for years. When you first started at West End, you came to my office, introduced yourself, and said you hoped to be a flight-nurse on my team within two years. I tried kicking you out, but you came back. All the time. You weren't kidding then. I hope you're kidding now."

"No. I'm not. And I'm sorry, Blake. You worked hard for me, and I can't tell you how much it means to me. But I'd never be able to live with myself if I don't fulfill my obligations at Adventura. And you wouldn't want a nurse on your team that didn't live up to her word, right?"

A long stretch of silence swelled between us. Blake ran a hand through his hair with a heavy sigh, making it stand up on end.

"Wow, Meg. I don't know what to say. This came out of nowhere."

"I know. And I'm sorry."

He stared at me, long and hard. A thousand thoughts seemed to fill his gaze. Questions. Doubts. Frustration. Curiosity. He mirrored my own feelings, which moved like the wings of a hummingbird.

"I know you are," he finally said. "And although I don't like this, I can at least respect what you're doing."

A deep sense of relief and mourning washed over me. Not taking this offer from Blake effectively cut my ties with West End Flight Team. Refusing the golden chalice meant I wouldn't get another chance here. But maybe I didn't want tired West End as much anymore.

He stood, hand extended, a wan smile on his face. I followed suit, accepting his firm handshake with one of my own.

"Thanks, Blake."

"Best of luck to you, Megan Bailey. You're a good woman. Whatever you do, you'll kill it."

My hand fell back to my side. The consolation of doing the right thing—even while losing the thing I'd wanted—filled the empty hole in my chest. With one last glance over my shoulder, I stepped outside his office and let the door close behind me.

~

Megan: Rachelle, are you busy? Can I stop by your work?

Rachelle: YAS! I'm ssssoooooooo bored. My client is asleep. AGAIN. I'm playing checkers by myself now.

Megan: I need to ask you a massive favor.

Rachelle: You're going back to Adventura, aren't you?

Megan: Yeah.

Rachelle: Come on by. We'll look at flights together. My mom will buy. You can pay her back later.

Megan: Thank you! I owe you BIG time.

~

"Hey Megan, this is Jodie Renner again. Sorry for the second voicemail. Look, we need to talk. Job opportunities aren't looking great, but I may have an idea. One that I need to talk with you about off the record. Call me when you can."

22

RESPONSIBILITY

Twenty-four hours, a last-minute flight, and a rental car later—I cringed at the $800 I owed Rachelle's mother—I pulled into the parking lot at Adventura at 3:34 a.m. An empty energy drink can sat in the cup holder next to the brake, covered by an empty package of jerky.

My hands jumped. My blood veins twitched. With this much caffeine careening through my veins, I'd beat Justin up Custer Mountain *for sure*.

Markedly fewer cars than normal filled the gravel lot. No lights dotted the landscape. I felt a nudging of hope that all hadn't fallen apart.

I stepped out of the car, enjoying the velvety darkness and the sweet, dry air of the mountains. Despite being high summer, a chill lay across the night, making me shiver. Without light pollution from the city, a dusky array of stars glittered overhead.

For the next thirty minutes, I snuck around Adventura, rushing from the car to the kitchen with as little noise as possible. An abnormal number of plastic bread bags filled the trash cans, and a few dishes were soaking in the sink, but nothing else had changed. I set to work. Simple tasks like cutting butter and measuring flour had never been so soothing.

When the staff began to stir at six, my plan was nearly complete. The sweet, sticky scent of warm fruit and crackling bacon mingled in the air.

When I scooped the first batch of crispy bacon onto a paper towel, Justin wandered into the kitchen.

"Megan?" His voice rolled with deep, sleepy tones. He stifled a yawn, eyes wide. "What are you doing here? I'm not dreaming, right?"

His sleepy gaze moved to the aggregated food near the rolling window. Stacks of golden French toast and a warm pot of syrup awaited. The door opened behind him, and JJ slammed into his back.

"Geez, bro," JJ muttered. "There are better places to—oh." He stopped, blinked, and jerked his head in greeting. "Hey, Meg."

"Hi."

His eyes darted around the kitchen. "What's going on?"

"I'm here to beg for forgiveness." I motioned to Justin. "From all of you."

Justin moved to the side, clearing his throat. JJ hesitated in the doorway, seeming to rotate through every emotion before his shoulders softened.

"I shouldn't have left," I said. "It was wrong of me to not fulfill my agreement. And leaving you and Mark when we needed each other most ... so I'm back. Hopefully that's going to be okay."

With his characteristic ease, JJ shuffled inside. He wrapped an arm around my shoulders and closed the distance between us. The friction in the air cleared. I wrapped my arms around his waist and blinked back tears.

"Food is a good place to start," he said, squeezing tight. "Thanks for coming back, Meg. We always love you. That was a ... messed up day."

The back door opened a third time.

"JJ," Mark cried. "I smell bacon! I thought you opposed it on twenty different lev—"

He halted as I stepped away from JJ. His gaze bored into me like a knife. My toes curled. JJ had always been quick to forgive, but Mark held on to emotions with dogged persistence, like Dad.

He swallowed. "What are you doing here? I thought you left for your perfect job opportunity."

"I came to beg for my job back. And apologize. To you and the staff."

Justin excused himself through the back door, leaving the three of us alone. The leaden, heavy air expanded again. Tears filled my eyes. JJ shuffled back until he hovered just behind me.

"I'm sorry, Mark. I shouldn't have left you in the lurch. The divorce frightened me, and I panicked. But still ... I owed you way better than that.

As an employee and as a ... little blister. Regardless of what Mom and Dad are going through, the three of us are, and always will be, a family. I'm sorry."

Mark and JJ exchanged a look, one that I couldn't read. At times like these, they seemed to be of one mind. Not a hint of forgiveness flickered in Mark's steely eyes.

"We almost had to shut down," he said.

I winced.

"Mom couldn't get every shift covered to help, so I had to draw up a waiver for parents to sign, saying they recognized I only had intermittent licensed medical personnel. Only five parents agreed. Five. I'm losing thousands of dollars because of you. You picked one hell of a week to bail—this was supposed to be my biggest group. Fifty campers. And now we have *five*. Now I'll have to report a loss to the investors, and I may not get funding for next year."

His voice grew in volume with every word. I held his livid gaze by sheer willpower.

"I'll pay it back, Mark. Every dime. That's why I'm here. I want to make it right. It'll take me a while to get you the money. There's this issue with a credit card and other people I owe, but I'll do it."

His bluster faded into narrow-eyed suspicion.

"Really?"

"Yes. This is my fault, so I'll take responsibility for it. How much have you lost?"

"Eight thousand dollars."

"Good grief," I choked, swallowing. "A-all right. I'll have to do a payment plan, but I will pay you back. I promise. And I can sign something if you don't trust me anymore. I get it."

His tense shoulders softened.

"Okay. You're definitely signing a contract to pay it back. I'll take it."

I motioned to the food with a tilt of my head. "I, uh ... made you a Naked Black Forest Cake."

He glanced around, his gaze stopping on the tower of glazed cherries dripping off gooey layers of chocolate. His eyes widened.

"'Bout time," he muttered. "I've been waiting for that cake all summer. Fine. If you want to come back, you can have the spot. But I still can't pay you. You'll need to hardcore grovel for at least a week. Make Black Forest Cake every day at dinner. Sugar cookies before bedtime. Also, Sione may challenge you for the belly-flop title back, and you have to lose."

His expression didn't falter.

"That's it?" I asked.

"Yep."

"Really?"

One millimeter at a time, Mark's trademark devil-may-care expression crossed his face, erasing the angst. He held out his arms. With a squeal, I ran headfirst into him. JJ and Mark cocooned me deep inside their protective hug.

"Welcome home, blister," Mark said, rubbing my hair with his knuckles. I pulled away. "It's always good to have you back. But there's someone else you need to talk to." He glanced outside. "She's been hanging out at the lake before helping with breakfast most mornings."

A deep pang of hurt raced through me. "Mom?"

"Yeah."

"She's here?"

"Until tonight. She has to work again."

"Where's Dad?"

"Up the river fishing. Took the whole week off."

I hesitated. Talking with Mom could go so many directions I wasn't ready for. JJ nudged me with a gentle hand, motioning outside with a jerk of his head. "You'll feel better after you talk to her. Trust us, Meg. She has a lot she wants to explain."

~

TEN MINUTES LATER, I pattered down the dock in bare feet.

A light fog curled along the top of the lake in wisps. Fish popped in and out of the water, sending widening rings across the surface. Tendrils of mist started to lift from the lake, extending my view to the reedy bank on the other side. Thanks to the low-hanging clouds, the day appeared gray and desolate. A familiar, lean figure stood at the edge, peering into the mist.

I tucked my hands into my fleece jacket pockets and stopped right next to her. We stood at the edge of the dock, staring into the murky depths without speaking. I wondered if the young moose would wander by.

"Hey, Meg."

I swallowed, grateful we didn't have to make eye contact right away. The words sat like a rock on my chest.

"I'm sorry I yelled at you, Mom."

"You were scared." She put an arm around my shoulder and pulled me close. "I completely understand. Besides, I should be apologizing, not you. News like that is bad enough, but childish bickering? We've let you down. In so many ways." Tears thickened her voice. "I'm so sorry."

I reached over and threaded our fingers together, then squeezed her hand. To my relief, the following silence didn't feel strained or awkward. Like the two of us, it just *was*. It gave me courage.

"Are you scared?" I asked.

She nodded, eyes glittering. The cut of her beautiful, elegant profile stood in stark contrast to the clouds behind her. I missed her long hair.

"I'm terrified," she said. "I've never been this frightened in my life."

She wiped away a tear with her other hand. In the distance, a bird called, low and mournful, over the water.

"So, what really happened? What finally drove you and Dad apart?"

Her shoulders slumped. "Many things, Meg baby. Many, many things. But I believe it started years ago, when you were in middle school. Things were busy. Your father was distant. He never opened up much even on good days, and that bothered me. But we didn't seek help. We just kept surviving."

Tears tightened my throat. All my memories would be different after this. I'd rethink every recollection. Every observation. A high price to pay for a once-innocent childhood. My thoughts shifted.

"So, it wasn't your job?"

"Not alone, no. Your father worked and fished, and I hated fishing." She grimaced. "The smell. Ugh. He hates running, and I love running ... so we didn't have many common interests. Anyway, I went into nursing to connect with people. Something I couldn't do with my husband. He seemed to cocoon inside and shut me out."

Already, my memories unraveled. Mom trying to find a movie at the theater Dad would watch, but never leaving. Long, quiet nights at home while she moved restlessly around the kitchen and Dad worked on his fly fishing lures. Dad's stoic silences and lack of conversation had always been normal to me. Comforting, even. But he hadn't been my husband. I felt a new pang of sympathy for Mom. While I loved Dad, he would have been very difficult to understand as a spouse.

"Then I realized how much I loved having a career," she continued, "so I threw myself into it. People *talk*, you know? Your father never did. I even tried to talk to him about fly fishing, but it didn't work. For years we grew apart. Neither of us stopped it. We didn't even fight—not until the end. Of course, my career played a part in the demise of our marriage, but it wasn't fully responsible, the way your father believes. I think it's easier for him that way."

Without realizing it, she reached up and ran her fingers through my loose hair. The steady movement calmed me. Finally hearing Mom's side brought new light to the situation. The hurt in Dad's expression when he'd revealed that Mom didn't want him—or so he thought. Like my debt, their divorce happened in layers. Layers of emotion that brought about terrible decisions. For some reason, that made it easier to bear.

"Does that answer your question?" she asked.

I blinked, peering into her soft eyes, still sparkling with unshed tears. I pressed my lips together, nodding.

"Yes. Thank you for being honest."

She smiled. "Enough about me—you're here. Which means you must have given up the job."

I pulled in a deep breath of fresh mountain air. The sound of the warblers waking up in the trees drifted across the lake. In the distance, I could just make out the vague chatter of the staff as they streamed into the lodge. Within moments, they would see their breakfast. They'd eat, jostle, and tease each other. Come visit me between meals. Request ten dozen cookies just for them and their tent mate. Try to put mustard in the ketchup bottle.

I couldn't wait.

"Yes. I did give the position at West End up. But that's okay. I think the hospital is on the decline. The corporation expanded so much that things have started to suffer."

"I'm sorry, Meg. You wanted that position for a while."

"Yes. I really did. But I think I may have found something else."

"Oh?" Her eyebrows rose halfway to her hairline. "Where?"

I grinned. "Montrose."

Her mouth opened and closed several times. "Montrose?" she cried. "Not Montrose as in ... but that's only four hours away from here!"

"They have a travel-nurse position open for an ER nurse. Starts at the end of August."

"How did you find out about that?"

"Jodie, a nurse recruiter I worked with, told me about it on the sly. Technically, she's not supposed to. But pickings back home were slim. She has a friend who works for the travel company, and they offer sign-on bonuses. I've already contacted the travel-nurse recruiter. My application goes to the hospital tomorrow. And they have a flight team! So I might hire on as a full-time nurse and work up to their flight team if I like it there. If I don't? I'll move on."

"Travel nursing," she murmured. "Now *there's* a challenge. New hospital. New city. New everything."

"I know! And best of all, I get to pick where I live." I squeezed her hand. "And for now, I want to be close to home for a while."

"But what about your townhouse?"

My lungs expanded in a deep breath. "I'm going to rent it out, furniture and all. That way I don't have to drag furniture around until I know where I want to stay. It'll be a source of income in the future if I ever lose my job again. At the very least, it's a place to stay should I ever find myself in this position a second time."

"So you're leaving all your friends?"

Moving away from the Health and Happiness Society wouldn't be easy. I'd miss them all desperately. But my parents' divorce had thrown more rapids into my course than I'd expected—ones I wanted to navigate with JJ and Mark close by for a while. The townhouse kept me linked to the Health and Happiness Society. I could always go back.

"Yes."

Her jaw bobbed up and down. Her eyes seemed to wrestle with something.

"Will that make you happy, Meg?"

"I think so. It feels right."

Tears filled her eyes. "Good," she whispered, tucking a piece of hair behind my ear. "Because I wouldn't want anything else for you."

The sorrow in her eyes opened a vein of compassion right in my heart. The burning sense of betrayal I'd felt at their divorce softened. Mom and Dad hadn't separated to hurt us. In their own way, they'd done the best they could. For now, I could accept that much and deal with the rest as it came.

"Do you think it can be done?" I asked. "Balancing a career and still maintaining healthy relationships? Do I have hope?"

She paused. "Yes. But I think it takes a lot of guts, communication, forgiveness, humility, and loyalty. Things your father and I struggled with from the very beginning."

My mind spun back to Nathan. To my conversation with Dad at Rudy's Diner. The happy glow in Mom's eyes at the hospital. Lexie's giddiness at her engagement. The way I felt hiking in the mountains when I'd first arrived. Saving Atticus. Working in the hospital during Gary's heart attack. Helping in the medical cabin. Mark forgiving me for leaving. And the deep sense of joy that thrummed in my soul when I helped people.

It all seemed so jumbled and slippery, like I'd never have a firm grasp on how to manage it. Could it all fit together? Somewhere in all the layers, there had to be some sort of answer.

For now, making things right with my family felt like the first step on a long journey of figuring out it.

Mom pulled me into a warm embrace. I inhaled the sweet scent of fresh cotton and let go. When she pulled away, concern furrowed her brow. "I'm ecstatic to have you closer, Meg, but what about Lexie? You love her so much, and now she's getting married."

Something uncomfortable and prickly moved underneath my skin. Lexie didn't even know I'd been home for a few short days. Thinking about her engagement still sent a twinge of pain through me. How I would miss her.

"Lexie has Bradley now."

"But she still needs her best friend. Every girl needs one."

Not after they get married, I thought, recalling the ghosts of my old best friends. "I'll talk to her, Mom. I promise."

Mom's hands fell away from my shoulders. Her eyes sparkled. "I love you, Meg."

"I love you too."

I wrapped my arm around her waist, and we headed to the lodge together.

How to Grovel to the Staff

- *Bacon.*
- *Cookie dough.*
- *Stop sneaking spinach into everything.*
- *More bacon*
- *Let them play with the grill. (Two minutes only!)*
- *Lose my belly-flop title forever.*
- *Clean the biffies for Justin again.*
- *Make Sione a roasted pig.*
- *Work again next year. For free.*

Three weeks later, I sat on the counter in the kitchen.

The gleaming surfaces, scrubbed to perfection, winked in the streaming afternoon sunlight. My nostrils filled with the tang of glass cleaner and soap. Outside, car doors slammed and staff members shouted as they loaded the last of their bags. Now that August had arrived, the explosive colors of fall didn't seem so far away.

New job willing, Justin and I had plans to hike Custer Mountain in the middle of September, when the leaves set fire to the forest.

"I knew I'd be sad to see the summer end," I murmured, eyeing the stove and perfectly seasoned grill. It hadn't been so hard to learn after all. "But I didn't think I'd be this sad."

Justin propped his hands behind him and leaned back.

"Yeah. Seems so ... empty."

Until next year, Justin and the twins would conserve electricity and funds by living out of the office. The rest of Adventura would need to winterize by the end of September. Rolled blueprints lay by the window.

Because the camp had almost broken even, Mark's investors had agreed to invest enough for upgrades for the next year. The kitchen would be the first priority for improvements.

Mark glanced around, his lips pushed to one side in a duck face. "Yeah," he said. "I knew you would be sad to leave me."

I rolled my eyes and smacked him on the shoulder.

From my perch in the kitchen, the windows revealed a naked camp. The cord for the flag banged against the tall wooden pole. Birds swooped by. Without the campers and all the staff, the empty skeleton of Adventura seemed brittle.

"C'mon," Mark said, hooking an arm around my neck and pulling me off the island. "You have a flight to catch and a house to empty out. In the meantime, Justin is taking JJ and me out to a really expensive steak dinner. Salad for JJ, though. I'll eat his steak."

My arm slid around his waist as he towed me out of the kitchen, JJ and Justin trailing in our wake. Trees swayed as we wandered through the camp, laughing. In the distance, the lake rippled in a breeze. With the scent of pine in my nose, I followed Mark to the Zombie Mobile, where my bags waited inside. The summer hadn't been perfect.

But it had been wonderful.

23

BEST FRIENDS

Three days later, I stared at a picture of cupcakes forming a massive tower in a magazine that Lexie had shoved under my nose. She'd always been so traditional. And yet ... so inclined toward cupcakes.

"Lex, are you sure you want cupcakes instead of a wedding cake? Didn't you always dream of a cake?"

"Positive." She tossed a kernel of kettle corn into her mouth and caught it. "Wedding cake is overrated. The English language doesn't offer adequate verbiage for my love of Oreo cupcakes. F'real, Meg."

A bag of kettle corn sat between us, kernels spilling onto the couch in Lexie's basement lair. On her computer monitor flickered the main menu of a DVD that we hadn't started because we'd been too busy laughing over wedding plans. With the help of the Health and Happiness Society, my townhouse lay empty and scrubbed bare, ready for the renters to move in the next day. A moving van took up the sidewalk and part of the street outside Lexie's house. JJ would fly out in the morning and help me drive to Montrose. In the meantime, Lexie and I ended my final day in the Midwest with one last sleepover.

She lay back on the floor, her hair spilling around her in a halo of golden waves. When I'd apologized after my return, she hadn't been as angry about me avoiding her as I'd expected. In typical Lexie fashion, she understood.

Still, a sense of hesitation held me back from fully enjoying the night. Would it be our last? Would Lexie forget me as all the others had? Lexie would move on into a new life this fall. I couldn't stop mourning it in my heart.

She looked at me.

"So," she drawled. "You ready to start your new job in two days? I can't believe it's almost the middle of August. The summer went by so fast and yet ... so slow without you to correct my dead-lift form."

I tossed the magazine aside and leaned back against her footboard. "Yes. I'm excited."

"What's going on with the credit cards?"

I cringed. "My first debt collector call came through today. But the sign-on bonus with the travel company should clear my account in a week."

"Urgh."

I held up a hand, ticking the numbers off. "Thanks to interest, I owe almost $3,000 to the credit card, $500 to Justin, $8,000 to Mark, and $1,000 to Rachelle's mom."

Lexie whistled low. "Geez. $12,500. That's a crazy amount."

"Tell me about it. The sign-on bonus will cover the credit card. The money from the rental will pay my mortgage, so I have to pay Rachelle, Mark, and Justin off slowly through the winter."

"Stupid adulting," she muttered. Then she sobered. "I'm going to miss you, Meg. I can't believe you aren't going to live here. Bitsy is hiding it, but she's secretly beside herself with anxiety."

A slow, quiet pang resounded in my heart. "I'm going to miss you too, Lex. You'll have a wonderful life with Bradley. I just know you'll be happy and have babies and ... you know ... move on."

She lifted one eyebrow. "I'm not dying, Meg. Grief. It's just marriage. More sex. More Bradley. Less Oreo cupcakes. Sad, I know."

"Right. But things are different when you're married."

"No they aren't."

Defensiveness thickened my voice. I straightened. "Yes, they are. I've been through this with so many other friends. You'll marry Bradley and slowly fade away. It's okay. It's kind of the circle of life."

She rolled her eyes. "Meg, don't be so dramatic. I'm going to marry Bradley, but I'll probably end up video chatting with you on the honeymoon."

"Lex, trust me."

"No, *you* trust *me*." She waved her hand between us. "This? This will never die, all right? You'll still be part of the Health and Happiness Society. We'll video chat you into the meetings. You're still going to correct my deadlift form, and teach me good recipes that I'll never fix, and make me laugh over bad date stories."

I snorted.

"And you'll be back for the wedding, right?"

"Of course."

"See? Our friendship doesn't have to die. In fact, it won't die. I won't let you kill it. I'll keep this sucker alive even if it's miserable. *That's* how good of a friend I am."

She smirked, her arms folded across her chest.

"But—"

"There is no *but*. I'm not the others! We're best friends. We'll make it through. Don't put their mistakes on me."

Hope welled up within me. Could Lexie and I still maintain what we had now? Could it be true? Oh, how I wanted it to be! One glimpse into her wide, determined blue eyes set me at ease. *Yes*, I thought. We could.

And we absolutely would.

"Okay," I drawled. "We'll still be best friends."

She scoffed. "Uh, yeah. You aren't getting rid of me that easily, Bailey. I'm like a friggin' leech. Got it?"

I grinned. "Got it."

Seeming satisfied, she reached for another kernel of kettle corn. Her eyebrows waggled. "And Justin? What about him? How have we not talked about him yet?"

Feigning nonchalance, I grabbed another handful of popped corn. "What about him?"

She rolled her eyes. "When are you going to date him?"

"Who said I was going to date him?"

"The gods of dating. They talk to me."

"Tell them they suck."

She tilted her head back and shook her fists at the sky. "Why are you so stubborn? You know what I mean! I know he's been in touch with you. I caught you video chatting with him before we finished packing your closet last night. Don't try to deny it!"

I laughed. "Hiking plans, that's all. This is critical stuff, Lex. I have to know what kind of hiker he is before I can even think about a date."

She pointed at me. "You still have to beat him up Custer Mountain, right?"

"Obviously."

"Fine." She sighed. "I'll wait for your love story to come together. But I'll be *very* impatient."

"Yeah, me too." I leaned back against the headrest. "Start the movie! Only Gerard Butler can croon about the music of the night."

"My pleasure," she said, clicking the computer with a wicked grin. "My pleasure, indeed."

YOU'LL NEVER KNOW

Hey there !

Thank you *so much* for reading Megan's book—I hope you loved it as much as I did.

That squirrel in the kitchen! I'm still giggling.

Rachelle is up next—and of course—I have a sneak peek for you below.

You'll Never Know

Chapter 1

Shattered Euphoria

The lemony tinge of cleaner embraced me the moment I walked into the gym. Home. My castle. The place where I escaped all my troubles.

The cardio room beckoned like a siren song. *Come,* it said. *Start your day by running all your cares away.*

Matt Damon would await me on screen. No, if I was lucky ... Gerard Butler. My calories burn would skyrocket as I jogged on one of many treadmills sprawled in front of the big-screen TV. Something about losing myself in the pump and burn and flickering lights drew me in.

Ah, euphoria.

Kellie, a girl with bright freckles and gobs of curly auburn hair, smiled when my best friend Lexie and I approached the main desk.

"Hey Rachelle," Kellie called. "How's marathon training?"

"Did my first twelve-miler last night." I held up a fist and shoved through the metallic turnstile. "Nailed it."

"So jealous. Hey Lexie!"

Lexie beamed. "Hey!" Her expression brightened. "It's not free pizza day, is it?"

"Nope."

"Bad idea anyway," Lexie muttered as she pushed into the gym. "Seriously. Who serves pizza at the gym?"

"You love it," I quipped.

Lexie tilted her head back with a sigh. "I know. I *know*."

"Wedding go okay?" Kellie asked.

"Yes," Lexie said. "It was awesome. But I can't lie—it feels good to be back. I'm sad this will be the last time I work out here."

Kellie's lips turned down. "That sucks!"

"I know!"

My throat tightened. "Yeah. Let's go."

After a quick wave, Lexie and I strode past lines of ellipticals and weight-lifting machines, headed for the changing room. "So?" I drawled, nudging her in the ribs with an elbow. "Tell me everything. We haven't gotten to talk since Bradley whisked you away. How was the honeymoon?"

Her pale cheeks bloomed. "Fine!"

"Fine. Sure."

"I never imagined myself a sit-in-a-cabin-in-the-middle-of-the-forest-for-a-week kind of gal, but it was pretty great. I can see why Megan's obsessed with mountains. I mean, I could never live there. Access to life was severely limited. Still. The quiet was nice."

"Did you even leave the cabin?"

"Yes!" she cried a tad too high. "Just ... not as much as I would have under ... you know. Other circumstances. In my defense, it rained. A lot."

"I'm sure Bradley was disappointed."

"Not in the least."

I cast her a sidelong glance, but she had her eyes trained ahead with unusual alacrity. Sweet, innocent Lexie had always been the frosting to my brownies. While I had flaunted my extreme obesity and obsession with food while growing up, she hid hers. In her basement. Away from her perfect sister. To have her even *talk* about sex in public was a miracle. I pushed inside the locker room.

"Aaaand?" I asked.

"And what?"

"Were you as terrified for him to see you naked as you expected?"

The blush on her cheeks deepened. "Oh, *that*. Ha ... well..." She tilted her head with a sly smile. "Let's just say my, ah, *fears* of Bradley not finding me that attractive while naked were deeply unfounded. I may have been insecure about the size of my thighs and boobs, but he sure wasn't."

"I told you!"

"I know. I know. Now that I think about it, I shouldn't have put so much energy into stressing over it. We've been dating for almost two years. You'd think I would have learned that he loves me the way I am. Anyway." Lexie sighed. "In the interest of full disclosure, I ate *way* too many Oreo cupcakes. "

A laugh bubbled out of me. "Oreo cupcakes? Seriously? How did you find those out in the middle of nowhere?"

"Bradley made them as a wedding present. They didn't taste the same as the cupcake bakery, but whatever. He tried. You really can't go wrong with sugar, butter, flour, and Oreos, right?"

"Right."

She stopped at the second-to-last locker, where we always hung our bags. She already wore her workout pants and shirt. After all the times we'd worked out together, she still hated changing in a public space. I flung my bag into the locker.

"When do you leave for your in-laws' house?" I asked while peeling off my shirt and tossing it into the locker.

"Tomorrow. After I clean the basement and finish packing. We'll probably drive all day Friday."

Thanks to her recent marriage, Lexie had transferred colleges, sold her car, and started to pack up the basement. Peeling posters of Gerard Butler and glow-in-the-dark stars off the walls had given me physical pain. Still, I couldn't help but be happy for her. She adored Bradley, and he adored her. I pulled on a shirt and rooted around for my running pants.

"I can't believe you're going to live somewhere else," I said. "It's so weird that we won't be in the same town."

"Tell me about it. How am I supposed to leave my little niece behind? My sister is still a hormonal mess, although granted, I think Mom secretly loves it. And Kaylin is three months of perfect chubbiness. She gets it from me."

"She *is* adorable."

"I can't talk about leaving her behind, either. I cry when I think about saying goodbye to either one of you." She blew her bangs out of her face, then tilted her head, her eyes narrowed on me. "Are you going to run for three hours again? I'm fine with working out, but let's not drag this into torture."

My shoulders tightened. "What's wrong with three hours?"

"Chelle, that's *really* intense. Sure. You're the cardio queen. But don't you ever take a break?"

"Of course."

"Have you since my wedding eight days ago?"

I hesitated. Did *not* running on Sunday morning and sometimes only an hour in the evening instead of two count? I jammed my feet into a brand-new pair of shoes and tied them.

"Let's hit the cardio room. The movie is going to start soon. I think it's *Wonder Woman*."

She eyed me. "You just dodged my question."

"I made an observation."

"That turned the conversation away from your exercise obsession."

"It's not an obsession. I'm training for a marathon."

"That you quit your job at an accounting firm to train for!"

"I got new work! I still teach exercise classes four times a week."

"Chelle..."

I straightened and acted like I didn't notice the worry in her gaze. The three-hour run with her there had been a one-time thing thanks to a very special movie marathon. Ever since I started teaching Zumba classes a few months ago, I'd had to cut my running time. That day had been an anomaly.

Besides, losing over a hundred pounds in the last eighteen months didn't happen with short walks on the treadmill.

"Just an hour today," I said, straightening. "I promise."

"You sure?" she asked.

"Yes."

"Fine. *One* hour. Although, seriously, I had way too many cupcakes, and maybe I should do three. But I won't. Because that's ridiculous."

We didn't speak as I grabbed a towel and flung it over my shoulder. My water bottle sloshed in my hands as we slipped out of the locker room and through the morning crowd toward the back room. Being amid the quiet whirring of the machines again calmed my suddenly stressed-out heart.

Just an hour.

Well ... maybe ninety minutes. At most! My Zumba class this evening was canceled for maintenance, so I'd need to fill the cardio time somewhere else.

Lexie could handle an extra half hour. Especially with a good movie going. She'd done it before for me.

Two rows of treadmills filled the cardio room, which boasted sprawling TVs in each corner and mirrors along the far wall. We picked two machines at the far right. Until I dropped from 265 pounds to 175, I'd always hated the mirrors. After that turning point, I didn't mind them so much. Now they were ideal to track my form when I started getting tired.

"Sa-weet!" Lexie cried when the movie started—just as I planned. "Wonder Woman! Teach me your ways, and give me your thighs."

I snorted, and she let out a giggle.

We fell into motion on our separate treadmills without hesitation. Music swelled through the speakers in the corners and rippled through the room. *This* kind of thing was the great part about Lexie. Everything came naturally. She filled the silence when I wasn't in the mood to talk, and when she was too afraid of doing something, I set us in motion. Even though I'd lost more weight than her by far after we started healthier lifestyles, she'd never resented me.

"So," Lexie drawled, one eyebrow lifted. Her blonde hair swayed back and forth in a high ponytail as she walked. "You had a new date after my wedding, didn't you?"

I grimaced and cranked the speed to 4.5 miles per hour for my warm-up jog.

"Yeah."

"That bad?"

"Could have been worse, I guess? He wore suspenders. To a baseball game. Explain *that* logic to me, will you?"

Her forehead wrinkled. "The guy that hit on you at the gym?"

"Yeah."

"Weird."

"I mean, it was fine. But the conversation wasn't great."

"If a first meeting starts with the words, *Hey baby, I think you fell from heaven,* then I'm not surprised. Suspenders? Really?"

Normally I would have laughed, but today I just grimaced. It *had* been a pretty horrendous pick-up line. "He was handsy," I said. "He kept trying to touch me."

"Gross."

I frowned. "Yeah. It's..."

When I didn't finish, she lifted an eyebrow. "Yes?"

My thoughts whirled. Although I had frequent dates, and not the glamorous kind, when I weighed 265 pounds, I often dreamed of how dating would be when I was skinny. The beautiful men—that I hadn't hunted down myself—lining up at my door. The gobs of date requests at clubs. Not having to drag the bottom of the barrel for a night out when the loneliness became too overwhelming.

So far, that world had eluded me.

"Let's just say that it's good I won't have to see him again," I said. "I think I might take a dating break. I'm tired of men."

"I took one of those. For twenty-three years."

At that, I did laugh. Then I cranked the speed up to 6.5 miles per hour and enjoyed the rhythmic pattern of my feet smacking the treadmill.

"Right now? That sounds pretty great." I recalled the glassy look in the last date's eyes after one-too-many drinks. Overweight Rachelle would have rejoiced—a chance to score with a muscular guy! Suspenders aside. But now it was annoying. Like a gnat that wouldn't go away.

Maybe that's what Chris felt like, I thought. My stomach twisted, and I cranked the speed to 7.0. Thinking about *him* would get me nowhere at all. Instead, I turned my thoughts to the marathon. Pictured myself crossing the finish line, hands raised. Sweaty. Salty. Euphoric.

Right now? Nothing else mattered.

"Chelle?"

I jerked out of my thoughts to find Lexie peering at me, concern in her bright blue eyes. I shook my head.

"What? Sorry."

"You okay? You seem a bit ... distracted."

"Yeah. Sorry. I..."

"Everything all right?"

"I'm fine. Really. I just—"

A wolf whistle came from the other side of the room. We glanced up to see two men stride inside, shirts torn at the sleeves revealing thick arms and broad shoulders. One of them, a guy with a lip ring, watched me through the mirrors with a lurid gaze. My nose wrinkled. I'd seen him here before.

"Hey pretty lady!" he called. "Always good to see you again in those tight pants."

I turned to snap at him, but a flash of pain jolted up my right leg. I flailed, grabbed for the arm railing, and missed. The quick-moving belt shot out from under my foot. My shoulder slammed into the treadmill, and I tumbled off the moving belt and onto the ground. My right leg slammed into the wall.

In seconds, Lexie was at my side.

"Rachelle!"

I shoved back to my feet but dropped again with a cry. White-hot agony tore up my right leg, like lightning into my hip. Once back on the ground, I grabbed my ankle and bit back a scream.

"Okay," Lexie said. "Oookay. You're not good."

I gritted my teeth and closed my eyes. The *pain*. It magnified through my leg, prickling and flaring in tight spirals. Lexie crouched next to me. The two guys had made themselves scarce, leaving us alone in the room again. When I probed the smarting ankle, heat coiled back through my legs. The muscles throbbed, already swelling.

Lexie stared at my ankle in wide-eyed horror. "That looks awful, Chelle."

"Help me to the car," I gasped. "I think it might be broken."

An hour later, Dr. Martinez stared at my ankle through a pair of tortoiseshell glasses perched at the end of her nose. The skin between her eyebrows wrinkled, and her lips twitched to one side. Slowly, she straightened, causing a waterfall of ebony hair to spill off her shoulders.

"Sprained."

Not broken.

"Grade 3—which is the worst one, by the way." She pulled her glasses off her face. I let out a long breath of relief. *Sprained* I could work with. Broken? That was trouble.

Dr. Martinez sucked in a sharp breath. "I want to cast it."

"Cast it?" I cried. "But it's not broken!"

"It's as close as you can get."

"That can't be right."

She propped a fist on her hip and lifted both eyebrows. "Are you telling me I don't know a sprained ankle when I see one?"

"No! I just..." For a long pause, we stared at each other. I blinked. "You're serious. You have to *cast* my sprain?"

"Rachelle, your tendon needs the extra support. As it stands, you're on the border of requiring surgery. Did you hear that? I can repeat it if you need me to."

"Surgery?" I sputtered. "It was a little trip on the treadmill. Nobody has to have surgery because of a treadmill."

Dr. Martinez tapered her gaze. "I don't like this sass. You want me to call your mom? Listen, I know my job, all right?" She jabbed a finger at my ankle. "That's one of the nastiest sprains I've ever seen."

Her sharp rebuke properly chastised me. Dr. Martinez had been my doctor for years now. I swallowed hard. "Right. Sorry."

"Look, we don't *have* to cast it. I just want to stabilize it until the swelling has gone down. There are really awesome boots that are practically armored tanks. We'll do one of those."

"Listen, Dr. Martinez, I'm supposed to run a marathon in four months. Whatever you do, I—"

"Don't count on it."

"What?"

"Do you ever run outside?"

Taken aback by the sudden shift, I leaned back. "Outside? Uh ... sort of."

"Sort of?"

"*Some* of my runs were outside, but ... most of them are inside."

"On a treadmill?"

"It's easier to control my environment that way. I don't like running in the heat. Or the rain. Or finding routes. Do you know how hard it is to find fifteen miles of safe roads? Not to mention the boredom of a track."

In other words—movies ensured I didn't cop out early, and having the treadmill control my pace meant I didn't tire out too fast. The mirrors gave me something to look at too. To maintain motivation.

Dr. Martinez rolled her eyes. "In that case, I'm willing to bet that all your treadmill running has weakened your tendons and bones around the ankle. Predisposing you to something like this. So when you stepped wrong..."

She didn't need to finish the sentence. One misstep. One idiot that thought he could impress me by acting like a dog. My goal ... *poof*. Gone. The goal I'd been working toward for the last eighteen months. The one I had lost one hundred and ten pounds for. The one I quit my job and started teaching Zumba classes for. It had to be *this* race. The Crazy Cats Summer Blow Out. Rock and roll music, confetti, and crowds of people lining the streets. This was the only race that would prove I wasn't ever going back.

"There has to be something we can do to speed this up, right?" I asked when the silence stretched too long. A light *tap* came from the door, and Lexie slipped back inside, phone in her hand.

"Sorry," she mouthed, then stood next to the bed, one hand on the crinkly paper. My gaze dropped. The ankle had already bruised a bluish purple. The strange coloring didn't seem to bode well.

"Rest, ice, compression, elevate." Dr. Martinez glanced down at her clipboard. "And time. Ibuprofen, too, but we'll have to regulate that. I'm looking at possibly four months to weight bearing, then physical therapy to full rehabilitation. In an optimistic view, you could probably be running in six months. Realistically? I give it eight. Just to be safe."

Disbelief plummeted to my stomach like a weighted balloon. Almost two years had preceded this. Two *years*. Lexie reached for my shoulder and rested a heavy hand on it.

Dr. Martinez stepped back toward the door. "There's a chance you could impress me. You're young. You have youth juice. With any luck, you'll heal fast, the swelling will go down, and there will be a *very* slim chance you can do it. In the meantime, my nurse will get that boot fitted and get you on your way, all right?"

She left before I could sputter out another denial. I blinked, dazed. How quickly had everything changed? Why was life so transient? Lexie cleared her throat.

"Chelle?"

"This can't be happening."

"It's going to be okay."

"No, it's not! I can't run the marathon. I…"

"You can run it next year."

"It's not the same."

"Chelle, maybe this is a good thing. You've been *so* focused on this that it's like … it's like you can't see anything else. Maybe this is a good chance to step back and remember how to live your life."

Tears filled my eyes. "I've been working so hard! I … I can't just … if I can't run, what … what am I going to do with my life? With my time? I … I can't *not* exercise. I dropped out of college. My job is exercising!"

Another silence descended on us. The devastation, so swift it took my breath away, tripled in my chest. I sank into it, terrified by its power. What would I have to work for? What was the point? Where would I earn money?

Without that marathon, who *was* I?

~

If you're interested in reading more, you're in luck! You can get your copy on my Shopify store, Amazon, and at your favorite bookstore.

Happy reading!

And thanks for being here. You're perfect as you are right now.

Warmly,

Katie

ALSO BY KATIE CROSS

The Health and Happiness Society

Bon Bons to Yoga Pants (Lexie)

I Am Girl Power (Megan)

You'll Never Know (Rachelle)

Hear Me Roar (Bitsy)

What Was Lost (Mira)

The Health and Happiness Society Collection

Finding Anna

Coffee Shop Series

Coffee Shop Girl

Lovesick

Runaway

Fighter

Shy Girl

Wild Child

Smoke and Fire

Clean Sweep

Protect Me

ABOUT THE AUTHOR

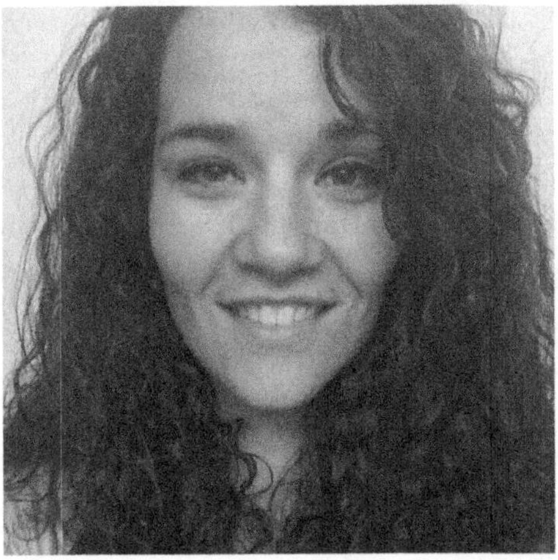

Katie Cross grew up in the mountains of Idaho, where she still loves to play when she gets the chance.

If she's not finding the nearest taco, she's probably hiking in the Colorado mountains with her three vizslas (you read that right), two children, and hottie husband.

Her favorite food is everything. She's a sucker for romance, though she seems like a toughie. And when it comes down to it, being present in the moment is her favorite thing to do.

To learn more about Katie, visit her website.

Made in the USA
Coppell, TX
05 November 2026

11315626R00135